# THE CHI REVOLUTION

# THE CHI REVOLUTION

## HARNESS THE HEALING POWER OF YOUR LIFE FORCE

Bruce Frantzis

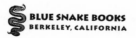

BLUE SNAKE BOOKS
BERKELEY, CALIFORNIA

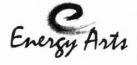

Energy Arts

Published by Energy Arts, Inc. P.O. Box 99 Fairfax, CA 94798-0099
and Blue Snake Books
Distributed by North Atlantic Books P.O. Box 12327 Berkeley, CA 94712

The following trademarks are used under license by Energy Arts, Inc.:
Frantzis Energy Arts® system, Mastery Without Mystery®, Chi Rev Workout™, Longevity Breathing® program, Opening the Energy Gates of Your Body™ chi gung, the Marriage of Heaven and Earth™ chi gung, Bend the Bow™ spinal chi gung, Spiraling Energy Body™ chi gung, Gods Playing in the Clouds™ chi gung and Living Taoism™ collection.

Lisa Petty, GirlVibe, Inc.: Book design and production
Richard Snizik, Snizik Marketing and Design, LLC: Cover design
Michael McKee: Illustrations and wave design
Damian Gordon: Scroll design
Abra Brayman: Dragon yin-yang illustration
Guy Kowarsh: Back cover photo

PLEASE NOTE: The practice of Taoist energy arts, such as the exercises in the Chi Rev Workout™ and the meditative arts, may carry risks. The information in this book is not any way intended as a substitute for medical, mental or emotional counseling with a licensed physician or healthcare provider. The reader should consult a professional before undertaking any martial arts, movement, meditative arts, health or exercise program to reduce the chance of injury or any other harm that may result from pursuing or trying any technique discussed in this book. Any physical or other distress experienced during or after any exercise should not be ignored and should be brought to the attention of a healthcare professional. The creators and publishers of this book disclaim any liabilities for loss in connection with following any of the practices described in this book, and their implementation are at the discretion, decision and risk of the reader.

Library of Congress Cataloging-in-Publication Data

Frantzis, Bruce Kumar.
  The chi revolution : harnessing the healing power of your life force / by
Bruce Frantzis.
      p. cm.
  Summary: "The CHI Revolution teaches The 15-Minute Chi Workout comprised
of movements from Dragon and Tiger medical chi gung. It also discusses the
major signs of depleted chi, eight obstacles to practice, current myths in
health and fitness, how to sense internal flows, and how to improve
meditation in order to access deeper states of awareness"—Provided by publisher.
  ISBN 978-1-58394-193-5 (trade paper)
  1. Qi gong. I. Title.
RA781.8.F728 2008
613.7'148—dc22
                          2007032961

1 2 3 4 5 6 7 8 9 / 14 13 12 11 10 09 08

# CONTENTS

# DEDICATION

This book is a culmination of all of the knowledge of chi I have acquired in over forty years as a martial artist, chi master, Taoist priest and energetic healer.

I thank all my teachers through the years including my last and primary teacher, the late Taoist Lineage Master, Liu Hung Chieh of Beijing, China, who took a Westerner in and taught him the secrets of chi, which had been closely guarded for thousands of years.

It is with my deepest gratitude that I extend to you this information to do my part to make the world a better place.

# Author's Acknowledgments

I would like to express my sincere gratitude to Jiang Jia Hua, who taught me Dragon and Tiger medical chi gung, and Liu Hung Chieh, who taught me the majority of the knowledge shared in my teachings.

Although several people helped in the actual creation of this book, special appreciation goes to three people: Heather Hale, Energy Arts Director, for personal, developmental, editorial and production assistance; Diane Rapaport, Developmental Editor, for her invaluable work in helping me present complex Taoist ideas in a way that is clear and accessible to modern readers; and Richard Taubinger for helping me conceptualize the book.

Thanks to Bill Ryan, Senior Energy Arts Instructor, for his contributions to the three movement exercises in the Chi Rev Workout™. Bill has developed a program for teaching Dragon and Tiger chi gung called the Moving Tiger Energy Exercise Method™ (see MovingTiger.com).

I'd also like to thank Lisa Petty, GirlVibe, Inc., for book design and production, Nancy Riccio for editorial assistance and Anastasia McGhee at Blue Snake Books/North Atlantic Books, Angela Hicks from the College of Integrated Chinese Medicine, Kurt Miyajima and Gio Maschio for support.

For images, design and illustrations, appreciation goes to Richard Snizik, Snizik Marketing and Design, LLC, for the cover; Michael McKee for illustrations and the wave design; Damian Gordon for the scroll design; Abra Brayman for the dragon yin-yang illustration; and Guy Kowarsh for the back cover photograph.

Finally, thanks to my wife Caroline for her copy editing and her never-ending inspiration and support.

# Foreword

As someone who has been working in the field of acupuncture and Chinese medicine for more than thirty years, studying with Bruce Frantzis has been an invaluable and amazing experience. Contrary to popular opinion, the knowledge of acupuncture points did not come from someone getting a thorn stuck in their toe and finding out it miraculously healed their gall bladder. In fact, chi adepts in ancient China were able to consciously feel and work with all the acupuncture points, meridians, internal organs and other structures in their own bodies. Bruce calls this making the body conscious (see Chapter 3). Not only can he do it himself, but more importantly, he has been able to teach his long-time students to do it too. Yet these are skills that most Westerners would consider to be something out of science fiction and absolutely impossible to achieve in real life.

## CHI GUNG AND ACUPUNCTURE

I first became interested in chi work in my early twenties, when I was studying acupuncture and Chinese medicine. Later I also studied herbs. The benefits from Chinese medicine soon became apparent to me and even now, I'm amazed by its power and healing abilities.

Over time I realized that chi-development practices could help me to strengthen and maintain my own energy levels when I was treating others. They could also help to prevent burnout. I recognized too that they could be an important health maintenance tool for my patients.

In 1993, my husband and I co-founded the College of Integrated Chinese Medicine in Reading, England. It is now one of the largest acupuncture colleges in the UK, offering a B.Sc. degree course. From the outset we were determined that students would learn chi gung "energy work" as an integral part of their study. After all, acupuncture is "energy medicine" and an acupuncturist treats by rebalancing a patient's energy. We realized that it is important for acupuncturists to have some experience of their own chi before working on others.

Chi gung is now integrated into the course, and we teach Bruce's system. This style of chi gung is gentle and never forced— hence it is well suited to the style of acupuncture we teach at the college.

Many of the exercises taught in the Chi Rev Workout™ in this book are fundamentals that our students practice regularly. One graduate told me recently, "I find chi gung helps me to center and prepare myself before treating patients and I wouldn't want to start my day without doing it."

## MEETING BRUCE FRANTZIS

My first contact with Bruce Frantzis was in 1998 at a seminar he taught in London. I had already read one of his books and studied with two of his certified instructors. Bruce was nothing like I'd expected—a huge bear of a man, very laid back, with a New York accent—not the typical "mystical sage" I might have imagined a Taoist master to be.

Then during the training he transformed into an extremely dynamic and powerful character, performing movements with a lightness and speed that surprised me. He demonstrated how to move chi in various directions so fast that he left me thinking, "How did he do that?" But I soon found out that he was always willing to explain. He loved to help us to discover how to feel and work with our own chi by breaking down the techniques into step-by-step practical exercises.

## A UNIQUE TEACHER

Bruce Frantzis has an encyclopaedic knowledge of all aspects of the chi arts and can teach them in a very pragmatic, down-to-earth way. His command of the Chinese language as well as Eastern healing and martial and meditative arts means that he is one of the few people who can truly bridge Eastern and Western cultures. Popular culture and the movies idealize tales where the hero learns to use some sort of magical life-force energy and attains extraordinary control over his body and mind. Bruce actually lived this dream. He had the vision and determination to spend more than a decade in China and five years in Japan and India, searching for and eventually mastering the energy secrets of the Orient.

By the time Bruce was eighteen years old, he had earned black belts in karate, judo, ju-jitsu and aikido. He then left New York for Japan, where he studied with Morihei Ueshiba, founder of aikido. Bruce was also a member of the university karate team that won the All-Japan Championships that year.

It was not until he went to China, however, that Bruce encountered the 3,000-year-old energy system known as Taoist nei gung. During more than thirty years of training in martial arts, meditation and healing arts, including working in Chinese medical clinics for five years, he was able to completely actualize the Taoist path of warrior/healer/priest.

The culmination of his training was with Liu Hung Chieh of

Beijing, a renowned Taoist Lineage Master. Liu transmitted his lineage to Bruce, arguably the first Westerner to be accorded such an honor. The rank of Taoist Lineage Master is one of the highest titles that can be given in China—the step taken after one has become recognized as a genuine chi master. Liu empowered Bruce to teach ba gua, tai chi, chi gung and other Taoist energy arts, including Lao Tse's Water method of TAO meditation, a practice which has been virtually unavailable to Westerners.

To date Bruce has trained over 15,000 students and certified hundreds of teachers in his tradition. He has a unique ability to share these formerly secret, ancient traditions in a way that is extremely relevant to modern life.

## WHO BENEFITS FROM CHI GUNG PRACTICE?

You may wonder if chi work is for you. In the seminars I've attended in the US and throughout Europe, people come from all walks of life and many different professions. For example, at a retreat I attended recently I met a doctor, a lawyer and a teacher as well as a truck driver, a carpenter and a Christian priest.

Also attending were martial artists, chi gung practitioners, meditators, bodyworkers, dancers, athletes, and many complementary therapists from all around the globe. They all knew they had much to learn from Bruce's system of chi development. Many other participants came from the corporate world, finding that chi work helped to lower their stress levels. The ages ranged from teenagers to those in their seventies. Bruce's chi work knows no boundaries.

## SOME EFFECTS FROM PRACTICING

Learning chi gung has also been a powerful tool for my own self-healing, both physically and emotionally. For example, before I started practicing regularly, my legs were very weak. I preferred to sit rather than stand and didn't enjoy walking or other exercise much. The weakness of my legs also meant that when I felt under pressure my chi tended to rise to my head, causing me to easily become tense, stressed and anxious.

Practicing regularly has enabled me to learn how to "sink" my chi to my feet. This has allowed me to develop far greater strength and stability in my legs. I now "stand my ground" much better in stressful situations and as a bonus I really enjoy practicing the chi movements. I have found an effective way to release the day-to-day stress of running a busy college. The chi exercises have also taught me to align my body correctly when standing, giving me better posture and freer movement.

When reading Bruce's book, *Opening the Energy Gates of Your Body,* I remember feeling somewhat dubious when I first read that, "the difference in body awareness between a paralyzed person and an average person is as wide as the gap between your present and future state of awareness once your chi practices have been established." I've learned that this is no exaggeration!

The exercises in the Chi Rev Workout have been effective for me and will help any person, regardless of health, age, body type or fitness level. I'm fifty-five years old and I can honestly say that I feel younger now than I did ten years ago.

## THE LOOMING HEALTH CRISIS

One of Bruce's main concerns for many years has been the fact there is an impending health crisis. Even when I first met him, this made sense to me—but at that time the crisis was only beginning. Now it is more obvious and what he predicted is coming true. It is clear that the West—both the US and Europe—faces a huge healthcare "tsunami," as he calls it.

As baby boomers age the population is becoming increasingly older. The boom has created a huge pressure on doctors and other healthcare professionals. The medical services of the US and UK are gradually becoming unsustainable. Statistics are extremely worrying. There are dramatic increases in chronic illness and anxiety, even in our children. There are shortages of nurses and doctors, shortages of teachers in medical and nursing schools, looming pandemics, and in the US, insurance, medical and pharmaceutical costs are skyrocketing. Many people, unable to afford the services they need, feel powerless and fearful.

## BRUCE'S MISSION

Since 1985, Bruce has made it his personal mission to teach people to take responsibility for their own health and help alleviate the pain and suffering that is already occurring. In this book he teaches us how to regain control of our own bodies and learn methods to participate in our own self-healing. We are the ones who can make health and healing our business rather than that of big business— countering the large corporations in charge of the healthcare industry. Despite the many drugs and diagnostic tests available, people are unhealthier than ever.

If we don't take control of our own healthcare, the well-being of people in the West will continue to decline. Are we going to just watch this problem escalate and let it swamp us, or will we react in time to do something?

## THE CHI REVOLUTION

It's time for a revolution. All of us can understand that health is our business and not someone else's. The revolutionary part is actually doing something about it—from the inside out.

Chinese medicine has long recognized that good health is the greatest gift we can give to ourselves. In Chinese culture, longevity and health are seen as far more valuable than money, success or power. Good health brings us contentment and happiness. Our physical, mental and emotional health comes from balanced and strong chi. The chi practices Bruce describes in this book are truly the key to health, healing and longevity.

Join me and millions of others who are taking back control of our bodies and minds. It is time that chi practices become national health exercises—just as they are in China. One way to begin to make this happen is by embracing the knowledge offered in *The Chi Revolution* and adopting a daily chi practice of your own. Taking this small step can lead to much bigger ones that inspire others to follow your example and affect global change for the better.

—Angela Hicks,
Co-Founder, College of Integrated Chinese Medicine
Reading, England

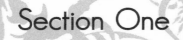

# Section One

## The Power of Chi to Transform Your Life

CHAPTER
1

# Awakening Your Life-Force Energy

A young man in his thirties winds around a slippery winter road. Suddenly he loses control of his car as it skids on black ice formed on the shady side of a mountain. The car whips and collides into a jagged boulder that propels it fifteen feet in the air and off the cliff into blazing tumbles. He counts six rotations as he is being knocked about in the shrieking crash.

The man suffered massive injury to his spine, with two badly cracked vertebrae, hairline fractures and several torn spinal ligaments and tendons. Each and every last one of his vertebra was knocked out of alignment. Three weeks following the accident, he awoke to the loss of feeling in his lower body. The accident rendered this once vital and strong man incapable of movement. The mental, emotional and physical anguish that ensued through his recovery is incomprehensible—unless, of course, this has happened to you.

Well, it did me. I'm the man who survived that horrific car accident back in 1982. It was a life-transforming experience.

My entire life before the crash had been about developing and refining my body as a martial artist—and I was proficient in the internal martial arts of ba gua, tai chi and hsing-i, as well as karate, judo, jiu-jitsu and aikido. At the time of the crash, I was the head of a martial arts school that I had founded after having studied for over twenty years with some of the most renowned chi masters in China, Japan and India.[1]

## HARNESSING THE POWER OF CHI TO HEAL

I had already overcome one life-threatening incident in my life. While studying in India in my early twenties, I came down with an extremely virulent form of hepatitis. In the hospital, doctors told me I was probably going to die, as had all of their other patients that had been infected. I healed myself at that time with tai chi and energy work.

However, back injuries are no joke. Doctors relentlessly pressured me to have a spinal fusion, which I repeatedly refused in terms that would not be appropriate to put down here. Given my condition, I feared that once my spine was cut open, the chi of my body would never be full again and I would not be able to do martial arts or, worse, even walk.

Miracles did not occur.

Instead, I did energy work on myself eight to ten hours each day while lying flat on my back in the hospital bed. After a few weeks, I went from being paralyzed to being able to stand up and walk a little. Nevertheless, the healing process was unbearably slow. My back kept destabilizing and the trauma neutralized every psychological control mechanism I knew. The emotional experience compounded by the constant nerve pain made life unbearable for me and everyone around me. The sudden loss of physical ability and the broken pride of an athlete left me in a profound depression. I felt I had nothing to offer my students or the world.

---

[1] You can learn more about the author's training in martial arts in his book, *The Power of Internal Martial Arts and Chi* (Blue Snake Books, 2007).

## OVERCOMING EMOTIONAL CHALLENGES

Total mastery of the physical body and self-discipline were some of the levels of my training while following the path of a warrior. What I had not learned to fully master was my mind and emotions. These were the more difficult challenges I had to overcome if I was to fully recover. I well understood the demoralizing effects of long-term negative prognoses and the morass of helplessness because, as a chi gung healer, I had taken many patients through these same emotions. I knew the patience and effort it would take to get me through the anger and fear.

In time, my chi gung and meditation practices began to help and I began to have some limited mobility. I added many other types of therapy—chiropractic, deep tissue, Rolfing®, acupuncture and massage. Even with these therapies, my physical abilities remained radically diminished and the pain always returned.

I decided that my only option was to do what I had always done when I could not find what I needed: I went back to China. My greatest teacher, Liu Hung Chieh, prescribed a particular form of tai chi and Taoist breathing and meditation. I practiced for eight hours a day for over three years. Much of what I did is still part of my daily practice. My back healed. However, as many who have had to deal with some kind of physical challenge understand, the principle barriers to healing were mental and emotional. When all of the constructs about who I was changed, the emotional traumas vanished, like smoke in the wind. My entire approach to life was reborn. My martial arts abilities returned and I came back to the United States in 1987 and began teaching again.

Today, my body seems to be a relic of the young man who rose to the top of the martial arts game. Although my walk might be closer to a waddle and I look somewhat like a big statuary Buddha, there isn't a whole lot that the average person can do that I can't. When I do brief martial arts demos in my workshops, many of my students report that they are shocked at the speed, force and ease with which I can deliver a strike while maintaining relaxed composure.

How is it possible? Chi. When using the arts of chi for external circumstances, the question is never if it is easy or hard; rather, with sufficient effort, it's whether the task is doable or not. The more strongly and more abundantly you build up your chi, the more strongly you ignite the healing forces within you. Today almost all of what I teach focuses on helping others work with the chi in their bodies for health, for self-healing and for helping to heal others using meditation and other techniques to overcome physical, emotional, mental and spiritual obstacles.

## CHI IS LIFE-FORCE ENERGY

Simply put, chi is the life-force energy that keeps each of us alive and connected to one another and to all other living beings. Chi is the life force in the universe, holistically connecting everything together as one whole. Chi circulates in all living things as well as in the sun, planets and solar system. Different cultures have given this life force such names as *ki* (Japan), *prana* (India) and *ruah* (Hebrew and Aramaic). The Bible says: "God formed man of the dust of the ground, and breathed into his nostrils the breath of life; and man became a living soul." The Taoists call the life force or breath of life chi. In many ancient cultures, strengthening the life force in a human being was central to forms of medicinal and healing practices. In ancient China, the Taoists deeply explored how chi could enable people to live well in the world. They created systems of medicine, medical exercise, divination methods and detailed pathways of meditation.

## TAOIST STUDY OF THE NATURE OF CHI

Taoism is one of the world's oldest spiritual traditions, vibrantly alive today. The word *TAO* also refers to the life path along which a person travels toward enlightenment. Many people know about Taoism through its ancient literary works, which form a practical foundation for all chi practices. These works also lay the metaphysical foundation for how chi flows through life and the universe.

The *I Ching,* considered the bible of Taoism, is a map that represents how the energy of the universe works. Discussed in detail in Chapter 13, the *I Ching* presents the Taoist view of the underlying nature and function of change, especially relevant in our lives today with the ever-increasing pace of modern life. Lao Tse's *Tao Te Ching,* the second most translated book in the world after the Bible, is the elegant, philosophical book about Taoism written from the perspective of an old man reflecting back on the lessons learned from a long life. The third seminal book on Taoism, written by Chuang Tse, is *The Book of Chuang Tse.* This down-to-earth book, full of epigrams and stories, often irreverently pokes fun at beliefs and judgments—spoken and unsaid, spiritual and secular. You could call him the enlightened hippie of his time. Both Lao Tse and Chuang Tse emphasize softness, the overcoming of challenges in a gentle, patient manner, like the power of water to smooth stone over time. These principles, along with the ideal of creating continuity between one's spiritual practice and one's real-world life, are central not only to Taoist teachings but also to the pragmatic applications of activating and managing the flow of chi for health, martial arts and meditation.

## EAST MEETS WEST

Many students ask me, "If chi has been studied for thousands of years and had so many wonderful benefits, why don't more people in the West know about it?" The answer is threefold. First, the Chinese kept these practices secret from Westerners and other foreigners, whom they distrusted and looked down upon. This went on for millennia. Equally, Westerners distrusted Asians and tended to discredit information they did not understand. Lastly, the

Chinese language was also a formidable barrier to overcome, one that few foreigners breached. Further compounding the West's disconnect to the East, during the Communist Revolution, many chi practitioners—including doctors and martial artists—fled the country. Others went underground and guarded their knowledge for fear of persecution. Luckily, many migrated to Europe, Canada and the United States and began to share their knowledge. Some practices, such as acupuncture, are slowly becoming accepted and incorporated as an adjunct to Western medicine. Yet, again, as these practices migrated to the West, the English language was formidable to some Chinese and, as a result, some ideas did not always survive accurate translation.

I learned to fully comprehend the nature of energy flow by living in China for over a decade. Learning to speak Chinese fluently was essential to my capability to study with many renowned Taoist martial arts masters, medical healers and priests. I also worked for ten years as both an apprentice and a chi gung healer in Chinese medical clinics. Throughout this personal odyssey, I was continually tested and given challenges, including learning to harness the power of chi to heal myself.

## AWAKENING YOUR CHI

Awakening your chi is a gradual progression that starts with becoming aware of the chi in your body, and progresses to understanding how it is connected to your mind, emotions and, eventually, if you decide to pursue a spiritual quest, to your spirit. Instead of being fragmented, all of your parts—mind, body and spirit—begin to profoundly connect into one cohesive, integrated whole through chi practices.

One of the greatest secrets of chi practices is that, no matter what your age or health condition when you start, you can improve and keep improving. Not only can you slow down the aging process, but you can also reverse its effects, because these techniques develop longevity and vitality. Once you learn more about how chi flows and works in such practices as tai chi, chi gung, TAO yoga, martial arts and meditation, you can integrate chi principles into your current exercise routines—yoga, walking, sports or performing. As you activate and channel the chi inside yourself, you will dramatically increase the quality of your life and become a pioneer in helping the rest of the world do the same.

## THE CHI REVOLUTION IS AN INNER REVOLUTION

Today, interest in and knowledge about the science of chi is reaching a critical mass in the West, a tipping point. The beginning of a profound revolution has been ignited that will transform the way we think and feel about health, aging and our relationships to each other and to the natural environment.

This is an inner revolution because it has to take place inside you. The only way you can develop the full potential of chi inside yourself is through direct experience and practice. You cannot just think about it. Thinking only keeps concepts as abstract thought forms. You may know that water exists and can relieve your thirst, but this is not the same as quenching your thirst with a drink.

We all have opportunities to open our spirits, hearts and minds. We all can begin an inner exploration to harness the chi flowing inside and through us. Welcome to the Chi Revolution.

# CHAPTER 2

# Creating Your Own
# Inner Revolution

M any people today are dominated by their emotions, thoughts, perceptions and mental constructs. Many others are in pain, suffering from chronic illness and disease, or leading lives that make them stressed out and anxious. They would like nothing more than to be free of malaise and to escape to a safe, peaceful place.

But what exactly does that mean? Meditation traditions like Taoism and Buddhism don't discuss freedom from the weather or from war. They use terms like "emptiness" and "stillness." What they mean by this is letting go of the obsessions, thoughts and emotions that bind us in knots. They are talking about internal freedom. There is no human being who does not have the need for internal freedom. You don't have to be thrown into the grips of a life or death situation, as I was with my car accident to draw a line in the sand and make a concerted change toward joy and clarity. However, you do need to know how to cultivate these aspirations inside yourself.

## MOVING TOWARD LIFE OR DEATH

According to ancient Taoist wisdom, our lives move in only one of two directions: toward life or toward death. Life is never static; it always tends to move in one direction or the other: toward order or disorder, balance or imbalance, coherence or incoherence, love or hate. The questions are these: Can you feel a sense of the energy of life inside you? Can you find the universal love that actually moves through life in all and everything? We must recognize that answering these two questions—instead of chasing the abstract ideas we hold in our minds—is crucially important to our life paths.

Once you find this internal energy, you will bring more life into your relationships, work and daily activities. Sharing the life force is what brings people together in community; with it, love and compassion naturally flow. This is why chi is commonly called the "force of life." When you have more life, you feel vital. Your life force allows you to align with life's natural, spontaneous rhythms.

## THE GREAT SHIFT

If you want to be free and move strongly toward life, a great internal shift must take place. The Chi Revolution asks you to get out of your head and into your body. In many people, the capacity to go from an external orientation of life to an internal one is severely blocked. Others in the West are waking up to the fact that no amount of external validation—material assets, status, affirmation of others—has ever done much to foster inner peace for more than a few fleeting moments.

Tuning into your inner world will not necessarily give you the instant gratification that the external world constantly promises. It is a process of becoming whole again, rather than a jumble of disconnected parts without any rhythm or harmony in relation to ourselves and those around us. The journey begins by aspiring to strongly feel and activate your chi, the key ingredient linking your body, mind and spirit.

When asked what truly matters to them in their lives, a thousand people respond in a remarkably similar way. They talk about loved ones, animals and nature—predominantly living beings with a life force. Nevertheless, this emphasis is still on the external world more so than on their inner worlds. The link between feeling better inside and having a happier life with loved ones has eluded them. When you experience life through your body, you feel all of the positive emotions within and can naturally express them. Thus, the extent to which you can fully engage with life depends on being able to fully feel inside your body and open up its energetic gateways. As you get your chi going strongly, your capacity for harnessing genuine joy and happiness will naturally arise.

## FACING A CAVEMAN

While in India, I decided to live in a cave for ten months. I was studying meditation and wanted to be completely alone to practice. It was the thing to do at the time, so I hired an aimiable gentleman to bring me food twice a day. Besides his visits, I was alone with little more than the natural rhythms of light and darkness twenty-four hours a day, week after week, month after month. The lessons I learned in the cave were priceless. What I found was that I had to face myself and the silence.

Why is it that people can go into a cave and live there for many years, yet feel incredibly alive when there is no one around and no external validation for what is called life? You could say it is because their lives are simple. However, as anyone who has lived alone in a cave knows, there are many hardships. But, at some point, I found I had something inside of me that made me feel incredibly alive and vital, regardless of my external circumstances, no matter how good or how horrible, or even uneventful. I found the sense of life inside myself. I was able to shift from seeing the things outside myself as creating happiness and love to knowing, sensing and feeling them inside my body at all times.

Fortunately, you don't have to live in a cave to have a similar experience. You can use chi practices anytime to go inside your body and feel what is real and not real—the forces projecting you toward life or death.

## FEELING YOUR CHI

Many people say that chi is not real, like a fiction novel. They liken it to old Chinese movies where dragons shoot chi fire out of their nostrils. Nothing could be further from the truth.

Anyone who puts in a little training time can learn to feel their chi. One of the easiest ways I help people to grasp the reality of chi is this: I ask them to lightly take the hand of the person next to them. I ask them what they feel. "Nothing" is the common reply. Then I ask them to remember back to a time when they were very attracted to someone. "What did you feel when you thought about them, when your eyes met or when they lightly brushed up against you? Wasn't there a kind of shiver that sometimes went right down your spine and even into your sexual organs?" This is your chi.

"Now think of someone you really feared or made you mad. When they looked at you or you think about them, doesn't something inside you clutch? Maybe your adrenaline rushes. Even if you aren't having the experience now, wasn't there a physical effect that came right out of your fear or anger?" This too is your chi.

The power of your thoughts and emotions to ignite a felt, physical effect inside you and others is also your chi.

## CHI PATHWAYS

Chi flows through precise pathways in your body and is reflected in the energy field that surrounds you, commonly called your aura. Taoist sages mapped the chi pathways and the main juncture points where these pathways connect over 3,000 years ago. The pathways are tangible and accessible like other circulation systems in your body. The realities of these pathways have become somewhat familiar to Westerners because acupuncturists use some of them to treat illness and relieve pain. Some of these pathways, such as the acupuncture meridians, lie close to the surface of your skin; others, however, are much deeper. The development of strong chi in all your pathways enables the systems in your body, mind and spirit to function at optimal levels. With training, chi practices will enable you to access, feel, strengthen and control the chi inside you. You can use these skills for personal health and relaxation benefits as well as to help others heal.

## CHI OVERCOMES SPACE AND TIME

Perhaps you know someone who had a psychic experience. Maybe they had a premonition about an accident or life-altering experience of someone close to them. Perhaps you've read a book or have personally experienced how positive thoughts can influence the growing speed of plants or how negative thoughts can make them wither, as laboratory tests have shown. Studies have even found that words affected the manner in which crystals form, which is probably linked to the vibrations associated with those words.[1] Perhaps some of you have been included in a prayer or meditation circle and were asked to send healing energy to someone who was sick. Maybe you found out later that they were better without any discernable reason as to how or why.

In all these cases, the chi inside you has connected with the chi circulating within someone else, overcoming space and time. Chi is part of the fourth dimension that is referred to in quantum physics. According to the physicists, in the invisible, subatomic world, energy connects all matter in one holistic whole. Taoists and physicists are in profound agreement about the nature of energy.[2]

---

[1] See *The Hidden Messages in Water* by Masaru Emoto (Atria Books, 2005).

[2] A down-to-earth account about how chi and paranormal or psychic effects are being borne out by quantum physics is found in Lynne McTaggart's book, *The Field: The Quest for the Secret Force of the Universe* (Harper Paperbacks, 2003).

# THE FLOW OF CHI WITHIN

Chi flows like a river through you, following the path of least resistance. When the flow of chi is free, open and unbound, it flows toward positive, life-nurturing forces. A strong life force makes you feel totally alive, alert and "present." You feel receptive to yourself and others much in the same way as a free-flowing river nourishes all life within it and the plants and animals that are fed by it. Chi is the force that links the circle of life.

However, your life force can become blocked. When energy is blocked or trapped, it acts much like a river where water backs up and stops flowing, accumulating sludge and gunk. If the deepest energies within you cannot flow in healthy, smooth and positive ways, they will flow in unhealthy, blocked and destructive ways. Where chi is blocked and stagnant, the circulation of other bodily fluids is equally diminished. If the trapped chi is not dislodged and allowed to freely flow, it continues to grow—gathering sludge and gunk. Its location in the body then becomes susceptible to stress, illness and disease, both physical and mental. Top-performing athletes are trained to quickly release the negative emotions associated with missed opportunities during competition so that frustration will not hinder their future success. They are practicing the art of letting go and releasing any buildup of stuck chi—a principle taught by Taoists for thousands of years. If unable to apply this principle, the athlete often ends up committing subsequent errors.

Chi practices teach you how to release the stagnant chi that builds and gets bound up inside your negative emotions, physical traumas, ruminations over past events and anxiety about future decisions. They give you the capacity to strengthen your life force as a counter to such malaise. They keep you vibrant and healthy for surviving the trials of daily life. The fundamental principle of acupuncture and all chi-healing practices is to strengthen and balance your chi by releasing blockages.

# IGNITION FOR YOUR CHI REVOLUTION

Every revolution challenges human beings to operate at high levels of potential—that is, to re-evolve. By definition, evolution requires and inspires change for the survival of life, inside and outside of ourselves. An inherent consciousness resides in all living things—people, plants and animals—to elicit everlasting cycles of adaptation. The motivation comes from deep inside.

Although revolutions are transformative, the upheaval the word implies is nonetheless accurate. You will not make this transit without struggle and some degree of inner pain. You will have to systematically reform the orientation of your life from being externally driven to one that is consciously, internally driven. All your facilities of commitment, attention, courage and intent will be brought to the fore. Socrates said that the unexamined life is not worth living. In modern culture, many have ceased to examine their inner world. Yet cultivating your inner life will set you on the path to a life fully worth living. That road is not a thousand miles away. In fact, it lies within you already. As your chi drops out of your mind and settles into your body—your heart—you are making your first definitive step toward internal peace and freedom and taking the path toward life.

The only one who can decide to take this step is you. By taking that small step, you ignite your own inner revolution. You become a part of the Chi Revolution on your journey to becoming a wholly conscious human being.

CHAPTER
3

# Making Your
# Body Conscious

L ove and compassion are the most powerful, unifying forces in
the universe. They are abundant inside you when your life force
is fully alive, when your body, mind and spirit are balanced and
when your chi flows freely and strongly like a powerful river. In
order for love and compassion to arise naturally inside yourself, not
just as an idea, hope, thought or affirmation, your body must be
awake and conscious. The nature of love is universal acceptance.
Love is cultivated as you find balance, stability and comfort inside
yourself. This means your physical, mental, emotional and spiritual
aspirations are being met and are in harmony with one another.
Inherent is a seamless quality between what is inside of you and what
is outside of you, a balance that is complete unto itself.

People don't make love to one another because it's a great idea.
They do it because something real—a spark—is ignited within them.
When the experience is genuine, a visceral, tangible feeling manifests directly in the body, surpassing any meaning the mind could
assign. Chi expands, connecting each to the other where the fullness
of their life force is expressed with an undeniable vitality. Born
from a biological drive, all living beings join in this union as an

essential to furthering life. Conversely, some find it difficult to feel
love or compassion because on a deep level they don't really care
what happens to them. As a result, they feel cut off from the sense
of life. They feel numb or dead inside, or they are depressed and
anxious. The contraction closes down the body, and the capacity to
care about what happens to others beyond a mental idea eludes them.

Socialization can go a long way to make behavior look pleasant
on the outside, but what's happening underneath might be a whole
different story. Inside, many people are dominated by the turmoil of
negative emotions and thoughts that prevent them from seeing
beyond their own agendas. These contractions take away from the
ability to feel and develop internal states of love and compassion,
which are not fed by external circumstance or by thinking about
them. Going inside and making your body conscious will develop
your abilities to free yourself from these contractions.

## FEELING INSIDE YOUR BODY

I remember my shock when one of my first martial arts teachers in
China asked me if I could feel my liver. I responded that I could
not. "What's the matter?" he asked, "Did someone steal it from
you?" He thought everyone could feel the inside of their bodies. I
didn't even know it mattered, much less knew it was possible.

A central goal of all chi practices is to train yourself to feel what
is actually going on inside your body rather than simply creating a
mental picture of it. We are born with the natural ability to directly
experience our bodies and the internal sensations through our
minds and emotions. However, many of us lose that ability even
before puberty. We begin the shift into living almost entirely in
our heads, progressively disconnecting from our bodies. In an era
ruled by machines, we increasingly try to solve problems with our
intellect alone. We spend a lot of time using only the mind, with our
friends, psychiatrists or doctors, trying to root out why we have
problems. Imagine if we could apply the same energy to actually

healing ourselves as opposed to talking and thinking about it!

*The challenge for people today is not to become more intelligent. It is to use our intelligence to focus inward and embrace the integration of the mind, body and spirit.* Sages in ancient China called this link the Heart-Mind, the awakening of true love, balance and compassion or wisdom.

## Get Out of Your Head and Into Your Body

Let's do something right now to consciously shift your patterns for just thirty seconds. Take three deep breaths, filling your belly with air. As you do so, follow your awareness into your stomach each time you inhale. Okay, your thirty seconds start now.

If you have just done this, the sensations in your belly will become stronger because you have put your mind consciously *into* your body. You have used the breath to connect with your body. This is what is meant by putting your mind in your belly. However, as you continue to read, you find yourself shifting back to *thinking* again.

Now, try again. Before you take a breath, think about some trauma, fear, frustration or worry that you currently carry inside you.

Now take three breaths and follow your awareness into your stomach. Can you feel a slight clench or tensing in your body becoming more noticeable because of the negative thoughts in your mind?

These two exercises, if you practice them, will help you make the connection between what happens in your mind and consequently in your body, and vice versa.

## Becoming Conscious

Biofeedback studies demonstrate that for every thought there is a corresponding reaction in the body, however slight. Most of our bodies are insensitive, unconscious and disconnected from our minds like inanimate objects we carry around. They don't seem to have anything to do with our emotions or mental thoughts. Although research has repeatedly linked stress and disease, most people don't quite comprehend the intrinsic connection between the mind and body. Of course, there is also integration of the spirit. Western culture does not acknowledge that the way chi flows inside us has everything to do with the chronic illnesses and diseases that manifest in our bodies.

Thousands of years ago, the ancient Taoists recognized the tendency toward relying on the intellect alone, a tendency that would create a fatal disconnect between the mind and body. They devised chi practices to systematically heal and teach people to sense the internal workings of their bodies. They found it important to recognize where chi was flowing or blocked, and to begin to free what had bound them, made them ill or stressed them out. The process is called making the body conscious.

## Training Your Internal Awareness

The ancient Taoists took a pragmatic approach to waking up the body. They started by focusing on gross sensations in their bodies and then progressed to the subtle ones. They advised doing what was easy first and saving what was hard for later.

Most of you have had the discomfort of experiencing a pounding headache at some point in your lives. More subtle is to feel how the headache causes the muscles of your brow to pull tight and furrow. More subtle is becoming aware that your headache gives you sour, negative feelings. More subtle is how the headache triggers other areas of your body, such as your neck and shoulders, to become tense. More subtle is to feel how the headache locks up the circulation of fluids inside your body. More subtle yet is to recognize the blocked chi of the physical, mental and emotional feelings you encounter and to use one of the chi practices to mitigate them.

# THE EIGHT ENERGY BODIES

Now many people, even those who can feel chi directly, associate chi with just their physical body. However, your body does not only have one energy field. The Taoists found, after thousands of years of research, that we possess eight different energy bodies that spiral into the energies of the universe. They can be likened to the rings of water that disperse outward when you throw a stone into a lake. Chi flows through each of the eight energy bodies, which vibrate at increasingly higher frequencies inside you. The energy bodies connect you to the same energy bodies that exist in all organisms and throughout the universe.

## The Eight Energy Bodies

1. The flesh of the physical body.
2. The chi body, which fuels the physical body.
3. The emotional body, which gives rise to your emotions, both positive and negative.
4. The mental body, which causes thoughts to function, whether with clarity or confusion.
5. The psychic body, which allows us to find our hidden internal capacities and helps our intuition or psychic perceptions become concrete.
6. The causal body, which causes karma to flow.
7. The body of individuality, which enables the actual birth of the full spiritual being commonly referred to as our essence.
8. The realization of the TAO or the entire universe, which few people ever actualize.

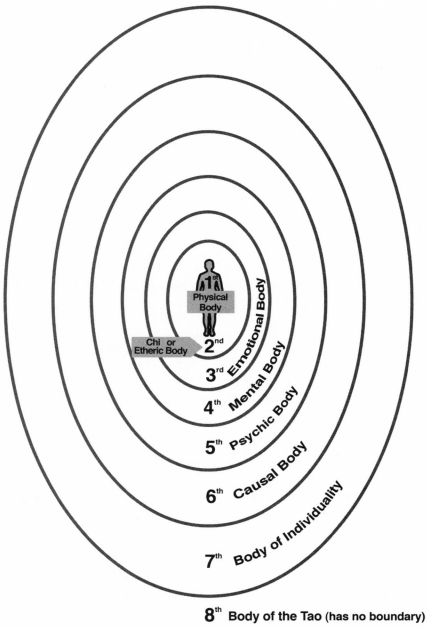

The Eight Energy Bodies

These energy fields comprise all the aspects that humans can experience regardless of time, place or circumstances. They are in effect maps that enable you to systematically become aware of the layers of your consciousness and the chi blockages they each hold. Eventually, the way your energetic field links you to the energies of other human beings and the universe becomes relevant.

Most of this book is about the first six energy bodies because they relate so strongly to harnessing the power of chi for health.

## CHI BLOCKAGES

When the chi blockages in your physical, chi, emotional, mental, psychic and karmic energy bodies are cleared out, they unite as one holistic force. In other words, you become a unified whole—one embodiment—as opposed to a conflicted jumble of parts ruled by one or more energy bodies while others are suppressed. In the spirit of doing what's easy first, chi practices train you to begin recognizing the blockages in your physical body. Later, you can release them and subsequently progress through the more subtle energy layers. Once you develop the ability to sense your physical body, you can apply your skill set to the ever-more-subtle energy bodies.

Chi practices were derived to activate the trapped energies inside you in ways that normal, physical exercise cannot. Energetic exercises like tai chi and chi gung help you identify, feel and discard what restrains you from realizing your full potential. The Chi Rev Workout™ presented in the final section of this book will teach you some simple breathing, standing and scanning techniques, along with a few easy movement exercises to begin training your focus, awareness and intention inward. These simple exercises— breathing, standing and movement—are the heart of chi practices. As you progress, you may become interested in practicing many energetic methods that are increasingly sophisticated and complex. For now, consider that to learn to read you first need to know the alphabet. You will do the most good for yourself if you master only one skill before moving on to the next.

Specifically, you'll learn some of the ways poor posture can block and trap chi in your physical body. You might have been told to "stand up straight," but maybe you've never had the physical sensation in your body to understand which adjustments you require. Poor postural alignments could come from slumping while you sit, which collapses your core; other problems include collapsed ankles and locked up joints, particularly your shoulders or knees. The initial lesson, therefore, will be to relearn good posture, which you can practice anytime, anywhere, and which will aid the circulation of fluids, such as blood, in your body.

Next, you will train yourself to focus your attention on only one thing at a time so you can recognize the qualities of chi blockages in your body and release them later. You learn to relax muscles that commonly hold tension, such as your shoulders, jaw or stomach. As your blocked chi begins to loosen, you start feeling better and have more stamina.

Many chi practices, including Longevity Breathing, tai chi, chi gung and TAO yoga (all discussed in more detail in subsequent chapters), release the chi blocked in the first two energy bodies. Simply put, they get your chi going. If you get no further than recognizing and releasing some of these blockages, you will dramatically improve your health, reduce stress and increase the performance level of your body. The subsequent steps begin to deal with how your emotions and thoughts impact the flow of chi in the third and fourth energy bodies. You begin noticing how your body feels when you have negative emotions and how you clench somewhere in your body, perhaps your jaw or stomach. The places where we accumulate obstructions are unique to the individual much in the same way we store clutter in our homes. You will need to find out precisely where your gunk has gathered before you can discharge it. As you begin liberating yourself from these chi parasites, you'll increasingly be able to release the obsessive nature of your thoughts. You begin to see the destructive quality of your turbulent monkey mind, swinging from tree to tree, compromising your clarity and ability to be present. You become quieter inside and calm the endless cascade of churning regrets, false hopes and worries. Thinking changes from fuzzy to sharp. Many notice that creative thoughts they believed were stifled forever appear with a lucidity they hadn't experienced for years or even decades. You begin to feel awake and have more stamina for greater periods during the day as your chi is permitted to flow more evenly and strongly. Higher-level chi practices teach you to clear blockages and wake up your chi in the fifth, sixth and even seventh energy bodies—intuition, karma and spirituality, respectively. A more in-depth discussion of karma is offered in Chapter 14.

## THE HEART OF HEALTH AND HEALING

The journey inward can take you into your body's deepest recesses. By making a significant internal shift in your consciousness, you will more consciously cultivate the forces of life within yourself. When your body, mind and spirit reestablish their natural connections, you gain the ability to enhance the flow of chi to virtually any part of yourself and to create within yourself a unified sense of wholeness. Cultivating chi is at the heart of ancient secrets for health and healing. Any exercise, diet, psychological or spiritual practice at its core affects your chi either positively or negatively. No fad or autonomous program of any kind will sufficiently guide you to an awareness of your essence. At the end of the day, knowing yourself will determine whether or not any behavior is practical for you, devoid of external influences.

Making your body conscious so you can become fully present and alive—in harmony with your essence—will be a design purely your own. Once you have it, the process of aspiring to an ever-expansive capacity for nurturing love and compassion for yourself and others will begin to flow naturally.

CHAPTER
4

# Self-Healing with Chi

One of my first acupuncture teachers in China, a surgeon, told me that after the Communist Revolution, China found itself with less than half of its former medical personnel, both Western and traditional. At the same time, the population had drastically increased from 662 million in 1960 to 830 million by 1970. Many were ill. Every day, the surgeon had 400 people in his waiting room. He could only see those who were severely ill or in danger of dying. He prescribed tai chi to all his patients, the most well known of the chi practices. He said he would only see patients who could prove they had practiced daily for at least three months. An administrator gave each of them a card, which had to be stamped daily by a certified tai chi instructor. Many other doctors did the same. Eventually, many of the health problems simply vanished. Noteworthy is that chi gung, elements of which are in tai chi, was officially banned during the Cultural Revolution and was "hidden" within tai chi and other martial arts programs so that it could be kept politically safe.

Today in the West we face a similar healthcare tsunami to that of China during the 1970s. As the incidences of chronic illness and other diseases continue to rise, health services are swamped and simultaneously become more costly. Training facilities are unable to keep up with the rising demand for nurses and doctors. The situation will only be exacerbated by aging baby boomers and their corresponding onset of illness and disease largely the result of unhealthy lifestyles. Stress is so pervasive that most people don't even realize the amount they've accumulated until symptoms advance to the stage of requiring medical attention. We need national self-healing practices to help us address this healthcare tsunami.

## STRESS IS KILLING US

We live in an age where the stresses on our bodies, emotions and minds far exceed our evolutionary composition because of the lightning pace of modern life and reliance on technology. Many of us are pinned to computer screens. Human beings aren't designed to sit, stare at screens and type all day, every day; we are much more suited for some level of physical activity than the sedentary lifestyles most of us live. According to the Center for Disease Prevention, stress accounts for two-thirds of family visits and half of the deaths in Americans under the age of sixty-five. The American Medical Association's statistics are more dismal, proposing that seventy-five percent of all illness and disease is stress related.

Chronic, unmitigated stress causes the body to overload, weaken and become prone to disease, a link firmly established in both conventional and alternative medical communities. Stress is the leading modern disease, evidenced by the alarming increases in heart disease, asthma, cancer, chronic fatigue syndrome, carpal tunnel syndrome, obesity and attention deficit disorder, as well as a litany of other problems. Stress is the price many pay for being productive, for getting the difficult, necessary things accomplished and for surviving the trials of life. The cost is our nerves, forced into overdrive, activating the "fight or flight" response, causing the release of potent chemicals such as adrenaline and cortisol into our systems. When the process becomes chronic by repeated activation, our bodily immune function is compromised. The energy that would go into building and restoring your body must be devoted to actually keeping you alert for economic survival purposes.

Your brain is a sophisticated sensory mechanism with the primary function of keeping you alive and safe by relentlessly striving to interpret its surroundings. When an external factor is determined to be a threat, neurotransmitters, the brain's chemical messengers, are secreted within milliseconds to send out signals for the body to respond accordingly. This is particularly useful if a saber-toothed tiger is chasing you. But our bodies react the same way when we freak out because someone steals our parking spot or cut us off in line—daily trials that hardly have any bearing on whether or not we will live to see another day. More alarming, this stress reaction can also be triggered by watching violence on television from the comfort of our living rooms, even when there is no actual threat at all. Eventually, if the stress mechanisms are activated frequently enough, your immune system is downgraded and your resistance to disease is compromised. A healthy and vibrant immune system is necessary to keep you from becoming more susceptible to the atrophy of healthy tissues, elevated blood pressure, infectious disease, muscle weakness, stomach and intestinal ulcers and a myriad of other complications.

According to Chinese medicine, stress depletes and weakens your chi. Tension prohibits your chi from flowing in a balanced and smooth manner in all your energy bodies. Stressful events have a cumulative effect, obstructing chi on ever-greater levels if not released. When your chi becomes choked off, you are less able to activate your body's natural healing abilities. As a result, you feel physically and mentally sluggish; you can't sleep; you might not be able to relax even when you want to; you find yourself holding your breath; you get moody; you feel revved up even over minor events; and, you generally get sick more often.

Maybe you can identify with some or all of these symptoms of stress, an indicator that your chi flow is inhibited.

## CHI ACTIVATES YOUR BODY'S NATURAL HEALING CAPACITIES

Everyone is born with the natural capacity to withstand stress and illness and to heal themselves when imbalances or malaise arise. When chi flow is low for whatever reason, your body's internal systems run down more quickly and your natural healing ability is compromised. Not only do you recuperate from illness more slowly, but you become more susceptible to future attacks. It is a negative feedback loop.

You can rejuvenate your body's natural healing capacities by learning chi practices, such as tai chi, chi gung or TAO yoga. You can choose to take responsibility for your health and well-being so that you don't become completely reliant on external drugs and treatments regardless of your age. Prevention is indeed the best medicine. Practicing the simple Chi Rev Workout in the final section of this book is one way of strengthening your chi so you can activate the process of self-healing. It is relatively easy to learn, it does not cost a large medical premium and it can start bringing more energy into your life before you can say "triple-bypass surgery."

## NOBODY IS GOING TO THE HOSPITAL FOR A RELAXATION ATTACK

The more you relax, the more strongly your chi will flow; these are key factors in determining your overall health and wellness. For many, this is a revolutionary concept because relaxation conjures up escape, zoning out with TV or some other form of entertainment, or taking a drink or a drug to "level" out. When people want more energy, they often think they have to rev up their systems with hard exercise. They think they need to pump more iron, run fast and hard, push and break through, go the distance. There's no doubt that physical activity is good for your body *if* it is done in a relaxed manner. However, when you overstrain, you activate the fight-or-flight response down to the cellular level. Your brain receives subliminal messages that you are in a life-threatening situation and the cascade of neural activity associated with your most innate drive—survival—is triggered. Tension is so normal that most never even consider that they could do the same activities in a relaxed fashion.

There is an alternative. We can overcome our conditioning by using our focus and attention to do our daily tasks in a calm manner rather than revving up. Then, relaxation becomes a living reality rather than a hope or metaphor.

Chi practices are renowned for training people to let go and settle down—physically, mentally and emotionally. As you practice, you teach your body what it means to release and systematically free up your chi in all your energy bodies. In time, you will experience deep relaxation and the qualities of calmness, awareness and inner balance. As your nervous system undergoes fewer spikes and peaks, your health improves and your overall stress decreases.

How many people do you know that have needed medical attention from a relaxation attack? Nobody is going to the hospital for a relaxation attack, and neither will you.

## THE SEVENTY PERCENT RULE OF MODERATION

One of our greatest challenges in living in a stress-filled, hurry-up world is the art of moderation. The central principle of all Taoist energy arts is the practice of moderation, which I call the "seventy percent rule." Now, I'm not normally a fan of rules but, in this one sense, most of us need to recondition our nervous systems to soften and relax.

The seventy percent rule states that you should only do any chi practice to seventy percent of your current ability. Striving for 100 percent or more inherently produces stress and challenges your nervous system to go into overdrive. At first, you might be able to get away with a stellar performance, but over time the physical, mental, emotional and/or energetic output necessary to maintain such levels will cause your system to downgrade. Equally, the body needs downtime to recuperate. Always driving in high-performance mode guarantees your engine will eventually burn out. You need to learn to give your body a break so that your nervous system can relax.

So, while you go about your daily routines and especially when you learn chi practices, don't push and go for broke. Doing so continually shocks the system, requiring more and more of your energy to maintain the same levels of productivity. Most athletes understand that fatigue and overstress lead to mistakes and injuries. Most people know that if they are extremely dehydrated, it can cause all sorts of health problems and depletes the body of the nutrients it requires. However, without illness, most people don't realize that stress and fatigue deplete their chi which runs them down, making it progressively more difficult to perform at optimal levels.

This negative cascade can be broken by adopting the seventy percent rule of moderation. This rule allows you to progressively activate your healing capacities without strain, over-exhaustion or damage to your nervous system. Moderation allows your body the resting state necessary to build and store chi, and it gives you a reserve of energy when you need it most.

Equally important, following the seventy percent rule in your chi practices forms beneficial habits of relaxation. You can also integrate moderation into your daily activities. These good habits train you to counter stressful events with a relaxation response instead of the brain's default fight-or-flight response. As you become increasingly able to engage with life in a calmer fashion, your capacity for mental, physical and energetic activities grows. Your system has the downtime needed to perform higher-level processes, enhancing its immune functions: regenerating damaged tissue, oxygenating cells, cleaning the blood supply and so on. It is a positive feedback loop.

# CHI IS THE KEY TO CULTIVATING POSITIVE EMOTIONS

Cultivating positive emotions, thoughts and actions when you are stressed or ill is considerably more challenging than when you are well. In fact, as your body tenses, your emotions and thoughts become increasingly negative. You cannot just wish away stress and negative thoughts, as many in the New Age movement suggest. Simply wanting to have peace of mind is not a long-term solution for overcoming stress because the body doesn't understand the meaning of your thoughts. The body just performs from low to high impact or rests, in tandem with another task or not. When you are stressed, the brain releases neurotransmitters to signal your tissues and muscles to contract or relax.

Remembering the good things that happened or are happening in your life, the love of your partner or children, or the beautiful places you have seen, most likely only provides relief for brief moments. You have to actually let go of what burdens you so that the chi blockage is truly cleared from the system. Your body continues experiencing stress despite the good thoughts in your mind unless the blockage is completely released. The more you try to control your negative emotions and thoughts, the more they will seem to dominate you. It is a negative and discouraging cycle.

Chi practices systematically enable you to let go of physical, mental and energetic tension while *simultaneously* reconditioning your body to relax into your activities. In the Chi Rev Workout section of this book, you will learn a short exercise system to develop your strength, vitality, longevity and skill for creating positive rhythms in your life. By remaining calm, you more easily handle the natural waxing and waning of negative emotions because you have the presence of mind to see situations for what they are instead of what you want them to be. Resisting or suppressing your negative feelings by saying to yourself, "I shouldn't feel this way," only enhances your negativity. You are left to feel worse; the tension has only increased. Have you ever noticed that urging someone not to cry often has the opposite effect?

Perhaps you already know that telling yourself you want to be happy does not work. Genuine happiness spontaneously arises when you are truly free inside. The heart of all positive emotions such as joy, love and compassion—universal acceptance—starts inside yourself. However, in order to be free once and for all, you first have to confront the darker aspects of yourself. In the immortal words of the classic comic book character Pogo, "We have found the enemy and it is us."

CHAPTER
5

# Overcoming Your Angels and Demons

L iu Hung Chieh, one of China's greatest chi masters and my most prolific teacher, once said to me, "You become what you practice. Practice suffering and you will get suffering. Practice becoming healthy and you will become healthy. Practice love and compassion and you will become more loving and compassionate." Many times, in order to survive and flourish, you have to reinvent yourself. The same old ways of doing things will only yield the same old results. Likewise, all revolutions have someone or something to overcome. Old beliefs and ways of thinking are reexamined. What does not work is superseded by a new understanding and a willingness to be open to possibilities not previously considered or available to you.

So, what does it mean to practice becoming healthy or to practice love and compassion? You already know that wishful thinking is often little more than false hope. You also know that your first step is turning your attention inward. Focusing inward will help you learn to recognize where your chi is blocked and eventually release it to get your chi flowing strongly and abundantly. For most people, negative emotions and internal dialogue have sapped their life force and colonized their bodies, minds and spirits. These are places where some of your blocked chi lives. They are the darker forces holding you back from acting on behalf of your best self-interests. They make you fearful about going inside to regain control of your internal life.

Chi practices are about developing a relationship with your inner self. The classic Taoist way of describing this is "relaxing into your being."

## BECOMING PRESENT

The ability to be present in your life is not determined by where you are or where you are going to be. It's about being awake to your experience through each moment without wanting it to be better or different. Many people spend a good portion of their lives fighting the circumstances around them; they want their relationships to be other than what they are, life to be better than it is; they'd like to twist some aspect of life into something it is not.

When you can be fully present to your experience, you see life as it is, without filters. You don't make excuses or blame others for the circumstances under which you find yourself. Now, you may not necessarily love the current state of your affairs, whether physical, emotional, mental or spiritual. However, when you can look at any situation for what it is truly and turn your focus away from the negative emotions, you gain the ability to change. Perhaps you won't be able to change the circumstances, but you *can* change how you deal with those circumstances. As long as you reject the state you are in, you lose the ability to change. Acceptance will keep you from becoming a prisoner that is tied up inside by your thoughts and emotions.

Being present is the antidote. The ability to stay present is almost completely lost in most Western adults. Being present enables you to regain the spontaneity you had as a child. Many of our relationships, even the casual ones, are governed by self-consciousness. Our actions, thoughts and emotions are governed by how we think someone else will relate to us or how we can manipulate others to think, feel, or buy what we want. Staying present depends largely on how well your chi is flowing. As long as you are dominated by physical pain, illness, negative thoughts and emotions, it is very difficult to flow with the moment, to be spontaneous or to have the desire and fortitude to change. You lose your internal power because the mind, body and spirit are internally confused.

## TUNE INTO BLOCKED CHI

As you learn to focus internally, you tune into recognizing the indirect signs of blocked chi inside yourself. In advanced practices, you learn to directly recognize the chi of the actual blockages, something most beginners do not need to be concerned with.

This chapter provides some examples of common signs of blocked chi inside a person, many of which I observe in my students time and again. Although there are many more, these examples will help you to recognize and locate the signs of blocked, weak and stagnant chi. You might consider if any of them apply to you.

### Pain and Disease

Few people today are completely free of pain and disease. They sap your energy of life, making it difficult to overcome adversity. However, often the impetus to change is when pain, stress and disease become unbearable or when someone gets a life-threatening wake-up call. The good news about pain is that it's meant to motivate you to take action. The next stage after pain is numbness—the surest sign of death. Better still, wouldn't it be extraordinary if people could shift to being proactive? You have the power to prevent most of the suffering and pain you could endure simply by not ignoring the warning signs. You must take responsibility for your health and well-being from this moment forward. Chi practices are not just useful in healing current illnesses, pain and disease; they also thwart future attacks by strengthening the flow, quality and abundance of your chi.

## Stress

One of my friends spent four days and dozens of pages listing the things that stressed her out. Just making the list stressed her out. Stress is a fancy word for tension. Tension accompanies most people like a shadow. Although there are infinite causes, stress originates for one of two reasons: worrying about the future or ruminating over the past. The more you cling to the past, the more fearful you become of the future. What was is history; what the future will bring is at best only a guess.

Since neither worrying nor ruminating can do anything to change outcomes, why do we expend so much energy fretting over what is? Mainly because we don't know how to release this form of bound chi. Perhaps the most difficult challenge in making the changes needed to release stress is that we feel so dispirited and demobilized. We would have more energy for releasing stress if we didn't use up so much energy worrying and ruminating. Getting rid of stress will help gently guide your attention back to the present moment in your life. Becoming relaxed and calm will give you a lifeline in a vast sea of changes and uncertainties.

The promise of the Chi Revolution is that no matter what baseline you start from, chi practices will put you on the road to relieving your stress and anxiety. You are on the path heading toward life.

## External Distractions

External distractions, even the most pleasurable ones, keep you disconnected from your internal environment. It is important to have the capacity to be fully functioning in the world, but continually multi-tasking—plugging into iPods®, computers, DVDs, instant messaging, cell phones and video games—is a common way to avoid what is really going on inside ourselves. Increasingly sophisticated distractions are survival tactics of the mind to keep us anaesthetized from dealing with suffering. Some pain is inherent in living. The challenge is to learn to not let it tear you apart.

Chi practices connect you back into yourself, even if only for a few minutes at a time, so you can counter the instinct to immerse yourself in external distractions. The sense of a connection to reality is not the same as bits and bytes of information and imagery overwhelming your mind. A random cornucopia of disconnected thoughts will not leave your insides feeling satisfied and fully alive.

## The Tyranny of Expectations

Many people are governed by expectations—what they should and shouldn't do, what they should or shouldn't have, how they should or shouldn't look and feel, and many more. Anybody who has been traumatized, mentally, emotionally or physically has a whole series of expectations about how life should or could be. When these expectations are unmet, that person has incredible negativity and resentment. When people play the blame card, it is about not getting their expectations met.

Now expectations are tricky. On one hand, if you want to take advantage of the marvelous scientific and organizational wonders available, you need expectations. The train should run on time, the television should power on, the car should start when you turn the key and so on. However, in your inner world, most of your expectations will put you in conflict with yourself and keep you firmly rooted in the past.

Chi practices strengthen your chi so you can break through blockages and eventually free yourself of the expectations that dominate your inner world. As you get rid of expectations, it becomes easier to strike a balance between your internal and external needs. Welcome to the present moment.

## Self-Dislike

Many people, when they look inside, don't like what they find. So many people in the West talk about self-love, learning to love ourselves, that it has almost become a cliché. A sad truth: many people dislike themselves. They believe something is fundamentally wrong with them, that they are unworthy. This might even include those who appear to be rather self-confident in effort to mask their low self-esteem. They bury themselves in good deeds or in their work. They use external comforts and even destructive means such as alcohol, painkillers and other drugs to numb themselves from feeling the force of their self-dislike. In effect, they're suspended in a fog, a cloudy haze through which they avoid the realities of their shortcomings.

The Taoists joke, "You don't have to worry; the moment you are truly unworthy, the universe will not let you continue to physically exist another second." The sheer fact that you are alive means that you are worthy of existence. Chi practices release you from self-dislike and help you reach clarity so you can deal with that which ails you. You allow self-love, genuine self-confidence and optimism to reemerge from the depths of your being.

## Difficult External Circumstances

If you have any question about whether life is difficult, I suggest you watch the five o'clock news. Doomsday scenarios keep us hostage to our thoughts: fears and anxieties about violence, terrorism, pandemics, global warming and natural disasters such as earthquakes, hurricanes and floods. This resonates with difficult personal circumstances such as loss of a job. Sadly, many people's coping mechanism is to just go out and do a little mindless shopping, drinking or zoning out in front of the television. We become immobilized and desensitized, and we find it quite impossible to figure out how to make a positive contribution, whether locally or even globally, that makes a difference. When we constantly focus outside ourselves for answers, we lose our ability to think for ourselves, compounding the challenges of difficult external circumstances. Eventually, this external focus degrades our inner lives. Our chi gets jumpy and disconnected.

Although you may not always be able to change your current circumstances, you can consciously choose to change how you feel inside. Turning your attention to your inner ecology for just fifteen minutes a day will at least help you lay down your burdens for a little while so you can acquire the tools necessary for change.

## Obsession

I once saw a bumper sticker that only used one word: "Greed." It reminded me of how many people are obsessed with acquisition and power. For example, many people have become addicted to gambling, which is about hoping for acquisition and power. The corruption that seems intrinsic in business, politics and entertainment comes directly from the mind being possessed by obsessions. The chi has become locked in the mental energy body.

Equally obsessive is wallowing in the horrible events of one's life. Bad experiences are a part of life. The really terrible thing is reliving those events over and over in the jungle of your mind.

Chi practices will systematically train you to let go and rid yourself of obsessions. You learn to identify what has become imbalanced before it gets so far out of control that you are overwhelmed and immobilized.

## Inability to Focus and Concentrate

In an external world that constantly bombards us with messages, input, noise, distractions and entertainment, it's no wonder our internal worlds get confused and jumbled. Very few of us have the ability to stay at one task with full attention. Sensory overload leaves your nervous system jangled and unable to concentrate. Since chi runs through the nerves, it becomes equally fragmented, inhibited and confused. To harness your chi and make it work on your behalf, you need to gather it inside you so there is one unified flow.

People who have lost the ability to focus need to be retrained *gently*. Awareness training is a fundamental technique of most chi practices. You directly focus inward, into your body, often on one aspect at a time. For example, the breathing exercises in the Chi Rev Workout ask you to focus on only your breath going in and out of your body. It seems easy enough, but most people cannot maintain focus for much more than a few seconds without their minds straying off track.

## Looking Outside Yourself for Acceptance and Validation

From the earliest stages of infancy, parents, friends, mentors and teachers have either given us positive or negative feedback. They either validated us by giving us love, acceptance and approval or rejected us with some form and level of abuse or disapproval. In most cases, they planted seeds that external validation was paramount to our existence and status in society. Many children are conditioned to prove themselves by external accomplishments— sports, productivity, grades—through goals and competition.

Now there is nothing wrong with learning how to set and achieve goals, provided we learn that they are not intrinsically connected to our self-worth. We are not our accomplishments. Too often, children are incapable of making this distinction because rewards and punishments are associated with almost every action. The result is that many children grow to be adults who have never learned to cultivate internal acceptance and validation. They are so detached from their inner worlds that they continue to rely on external confirmation and keeping up with the Joneses.

Your chi practice will help you develop the ability to assess your internal strengths and weaknesses and to decrease your dependence on external validation. The more you can get real with yourself about where you stand and what you are feeling inside, the better your chance to relax into and accept who you are.

## Inability to Be Alone with Yourself

When we were children, we didn't think about being alone. We found pleasure in almost everything we did; we took delight in learning new skills and we could do them over and over with great pleasure. We didn't even have a problem just "spacing out" and looking at the clouds or changing color of the grass when the wind blew. As we grew up, many of us lost the ability to be comfortable being alone with ourselves, with doing nothing. The silences around us began to make us feel ill at ease. Many of us felt guilty when we were not being productive, and silence tuned us into an inner world that made us feel uncomfortable.

One of the miracles of chi practices is that they give you a comprehensive system, a method that works, for tuning into what blocks you and getting rid of it. Then silence and stillness once again become magical and fascinating.

## QUALITIES OF STUCK CHI

The darker side of our nature has the power to illuminate the ways in which chi can be blocked inside of our emotions and thoughts. We first learn to recognize indirect signs of blocked chi and later directly link these signs to tangible sensations inside our bodies. For example, we become capable of identifying the energy behind our self-dislike or need for external validation.

Many students often ask me how stuck energy feels inside their bodies. There is no question about precisely where chi is stuck in your body when a masseuse finds a sore point in your muscle, tissue or ligament. You involuntarily curl into a fetal position and maybe old memories start pouring out. You might feel upset or actually start crying, screaming or ranting. However, some blockages are more subtle.

In my classes, I sometimes ask my students to strongly hold a fist for five minutes to give them a concrete example of what stuck chi feels like and how it has cascading effects in the body and mind. Typically, the students report experiencing any one or all of the four qualities of stuck chi. They recognize that it gives them a tremendous amount of physical discomfort and tension. They report that tension is uncomfortable and takes a lot of energy to sustain. Their fists and knuckles turn white. The fluids and the chi have flowed out of the hand and left it stiff and hard. The muscles and connective tissues in the hand contract and temporarily shorten. The feelings of tension and discomfort start traveling up the arm into the neck, shoulders and jaw, further tensing their bodies. Most of them begin feeling negative emotions, such as "Why is my teacher making me do something that makes me feel like this?" They learn that tension in the body makes for tension in the nerves. For some, the tension that travels from the hands may hit other blockages and might even trigger the emotions that caused the specific blockages. When they unclench their fists, it takes almost double the time for the chi and the fluids to flow back into their hands and allow them to feel normal again.

## INDIRECT BECOMES DIRECT

In advanced chi practices, your focus will take you beyond experiencing only indirect signs of blocked chi. You learn to feel where chi is directly blocked inside each energy body, progressing from the first energy body inwards.

Blocked chi has one or more of four qualities:

- o *Tension*—physical, emotional or mental; two opposites pulling you in different directions.
- o *Contraction*—constriction, such as the physical constriction of your muscles or an emotional hang-up, such as suppressing or holding anger or sadness.
- o *Strength*—the feeling of pushing or clinging.
- o *The feeling that something does not feel quite right, especially if you don't know what it is*—usually a nonspecific,

non-localized sensation of unease, discomfort, vague pain or just dead spots where there is no feeling at all.

When your chi is not blocked, these same places in your body won't call attention to themselves, nor will they call forth negative emotions or confused mental thoughts. You'll simply feel alive and relaxed.

## BECOMING FULLY ALIVE

Perhaps finding out more about your misery is not appealing. Perhaps you don't want to find out how your body has locked up, how driven you are by negative images, thoughts and fears or how much stress you carry. Perhaps you are not at ease with silence and being alone with yourself because you always seem to have a myriad of other things to do or other people for whom to care.

However, in order to open yourself to life, you will have to get through the darker side of your human nature. Taoists talk about inner demons and, equally, inner angels. Your demons are those things that you don't like about yourself and wish to change. Your angels are strengths that can become overdeveloped inside you and contribute to imbalances.

One of the oldest Taoist principles says that by paying attention only to your strengths, you actually make your weaknesses more severe—physically, mentally, emotionally and spiritually. There's no doubt that developing your natural talents in business is helpful, but your health is not a business proposition. Many of us have learned to use our strengths in order to hide the darker sides of our nature and receive external validation that we are worthy of existence. In this way, your angels may contribute to a diluted self-perception, which is the opposite of the clarity and balance you're seeking if you want to be happy. Chi practices teach us to focus and deal with our weaknesses so we can be healthy on all levels.

Chi is free. It's present inside you whether you can feel it yet or not. But you have to focus your attention and intention, and you have to practice.

Whatever your particular challenges might be, your primary challenge in the Chi Revolution will be confronting your angels and demons directly. If you can face your angels and demons in a detached way, you will free what traps you and enable the love inside you to flow freely again.

# CHAPTER 6

# Twelve Myths of Health and Fitness

T he running champion Jim Fixx is mainly remembered as the genius who started the fitness revolution back in the 1970s with his best-selling book, *The Complete Book of Running.* Fixx sadly died at the age of 52 from a heart attack. His arteries were plugged with too much cholesterol. Although Fixx trumpeted the health benefits of running and jogging, this high-impact exercise without any consideration of cholesterol resulted in some of the problems he thought he was preventing.

## SEPARATING MYTH FROM FACT

Fixx's story highlights one of the challenges in making choices about health, fitness and stress reduction. The barrage of often conflicting information from entertainment, health and diet magazines and, of course, advertising steers us toward practices that may not be effective or right for us. We try different exercises, diets, pills, and machines, and we keep moving along a smorgasbord of fads and quick fixes that do little in the long term. To add insult to injury, myths and misinformation about health and fitness are common in virtually all media. It is no wonder we jump from one promise to another, consciously or subconsciously adopting beliefs in programs that have little merit over time. The Chi Revolution is about life transformation. To get there, you must shift your priorities toward the life inside you. Let's take a few of the most common yet absurd paradigms of our modern age and see if any have taken hold of you.

## Myth #1:  If my body looks good, I must be healthy.

## Fact:  Health has little to do with a beautiful body.

Like a new car, you can look good on the outside and internally have parts that are weak and malfunctioning. You can appear fit and beautiful and not be healthy. You might already suffer from ulcers, allergies, asthma or diabetes. You might get colds often and recover progressively less quickly. You might be able to run five miles and do a hundred push-ups and still feel anxious, stressed and ragged out most of the time. Your joints might ache and you might have lower back pain that the chiropractors can't seem to fix.

By appealing to our vanity and fear of aging, advertisers persuade Westerners to shell out billions of dollars every year on cosmetics and beauty products, butt tighteners, abdominal workout machines and other exercise contraptions, get-thin and better-sex pills, breast enlargements and the clothes to go with them. Truly being healthy—energetic fitness—is not about how you look; it's about how you feel. It's about making your body, mind and spirit work together as a team.

## Myth #2:  Life is better for the young and slim.

## Fact:  Life is better when you feel good.

If you believe this myth, you have been sucker-punched by a multi-billion-dollar industry that promotes the cult of youth and slimness. However youthful and slim a person may look, he/she is increasingly feeling the burdens of low self-esteem, chronic illnesses, stress, attention deficit and depression just the same as everyone else.

Sadly, this myth is incredibly powerful. In today's culture, we idolize youth and make youthful appearance our highest good, our religion, our mystery cult. People approaching their forties—or even their thirties—are panicked about getting older. Baby boomers are spending billions on re-sculpting their appearances and the elderly are shunned by the young as pariahs of what they think they want to avoid.

When you don't feel good, life sucks. And when you don't feel good, the really great gifts in life—health, love, happiness, relaxation, spontaneity, laughter, sex, joy—seem as distant and legendary as Timbuktu. How do you get to feeling good on the inside? Try tai chi, chi gung or any other chi practice. It will give you all these gifts for the price of one.

## Myth #3: Aging is about decline and losing the ability to "get it up"!

## Fact: You can obtain health, vibrancy and sexual vitality well into your old age.

I remember when my own beliefs about aging changed. I went to Taiwan to meet Wang Shu Jin, a renowned master of the Taoist martial arts of ba gua and tai chi, who was in his late sixties at the time. I was a hotshot nineteen-year-old with black belts in karate and other Japanese martial arts and an attitude to match. My first view of Wang was of an older, overweight, round-looking man casually strolling to the park swinging two bird cages. As soon as I introduced myself, he told me that karate was for fighting old women and children. "I can eat more than you. I can have more sex than you and I can fight better than you. Yet you call yourself healthy. Well, young man, there is a lot more to being healthy than being young, and it all comes down to how much chi you have," he chuckled. Then Wang proved it by bruising more than my ego as he effortlessly knocked me around at will. I couldn't get near him let alone defend myself. It was the first time I understood that youth did not always mean power and vitality, and aging did not always mean decline!

Chi practices such as tai chi, chi gung and Taoist yoga have worked to keep people young in body and mind for thousands of years. They are often called longevity exercises because they are effective at restoring the flexibility, sexual vitality and stamina of youth.

## Myth #4:  Six-pack abs are good for you.

## Fact:  Tight abs can mess up your internal organs.

The billion-dollar industry that has you believing you need flat abs is part of the "young and slim" cult. What is under the skin of those oh-so-tight, flat and perfect abs can lead to big problems. Sucking and pinching in the abdominal muscles can foreshorten the ligaments that hold your liver, spleen and kidneys together. Eventually they could touch, especially when you move and twist, cutting off the blood supply where they impinge on each other. And those areas become just like the stagnant backwater pools where the river does not flow, a little putrid and disease prone. If you put stress and anxiety into the mix, those abdominal muscles squeeze even harder on those delicate internal organs. And guess where disease commonly strikes? Right in the internal organs.

Chi practices are about your internal health. They are renowned for improving the health of your internal organs.

## Myth #5:  Obese people are unhealthy.

## Fact:  Obese people can be healthy.

Health has to do with what is going on inside your body, not with how much you weigh. In our culture, obesity is becoming a norm. According to health researchers, eight out of ten people over the age of twenty-five and one out of five people under the age of nineteen are obese. The increase in obesity is being matched by increases in such diseases as type II diabetes and heart problems.

The good news is that being overweight per se does not have to lead to ill health. You can be fat and dumpy-looking but still have healthy internal organs, be free of pain and illness, enjoy a full sex life and handle immense amounts of stress in a relaxed manner. Our kids can be healthy too. Indeed, there are increased health risks associated with obesity; however, the larger issue is that seventy-eight percent of the American population is not meeting basic activity levels. That's a more shocking statistic than how many people are overweight. Weight is not the problem: the lack of movement is—not keeping fit, healthy and relaxed.

Low-impact chi practices are renowned for helping obese people stay fit inside their bodies.

## Myth #6: No pain, no gain.

### Fact: The more you push and strain, the more stress reigns.

"No pain, no gain" is the mantra of bodybuilders, salespeople, athletes and workaholics. Do you honestly believe that achievement is only gained by hardship and strain? This myth has been fostered from youth, when you first started becoming goal-oriented and measuring results by grades, competitions, status and the pressure from parents and teachers to "try harder."

Going for broke uses up your chi reserves, adds to your stress levels and incrementally weakens your body. By pushing to succeed, you increasingly strain your nervous system and depend more and more on adrenaline to keep going. Not only is this stressful, but it is very similar to the nature of addictions. You push yourself toward the next hit, the next high, the biggest adrenaline rush, the newest acquisition, the next of whatever hides behind the push. Strain is literally killing you.

Energetic fitness is based on moderation, increasing your chi reserves and giving you the stamina and vitality for almost everything you do. Supercharging your chi can turn you into a super performer with no straining necessary. Today, many executives are learning chi practices because the techniques help them decrease their stress while increasing their ability to maintain a high rate of productivity. Likewise, many athletes who commonly suffer from high stress and high rates of injury are learning that chi practices help them stay "in the zone" longer and keep them stronger. Getting more energy is about relaxing—not pushing and going for broke.

## Myth #7: Circulation is best improved by doing aerobic exercise.

## Fact: Chi exercises, done slowly and in a relaxed manner, are an equally powerful method for improving circulation.

Western medical studies show that the circulation boost for people who spend twenty minutes doing chi exercise is as effective as spending the same twenty minutes doing aerobic exercise.[1]

Although aerobics pump up the heart rate, forcing blood through constricted areas and flooding blood vessels, it is not enough. It is the equivalent of increasing the pressure to run water through constricted and kinked pipes. And if you add stress into this mix, they burst, just like poor Jim Fixx!

Chi exercises work differently. They increase the pressure within the blood vessels, thereby improving their elasticity, which leads to a flooding of the capillary beds. There is no pressure on the heart to work harder to boost circulation. Chi exercises have some cardiovascular benefits that aerobic exercises commonly *do not*. Besides reducing blood pressure, chi exercises relax the nervous system, which also helps all the fluids in your body to flow more easily. You exercise your whole body, so that everything inside you is equally strengthened.

---

[1] Young DR, Appel LJ, Jee S, and Miller ER. 1999. "The Effects of Aerobic Exercise and T'ai Chi on Blood Pressure in Older People: Results of a Randomized Trial" in *Journal of the American Geriatrics Society* 47(3): 277-84.

## Myth #8:  Relaxation is about zoning out and escaping.

## Fact:  Relaxation is about tuning into your body and letting go.

Few Westerners have ever experienced deep relaxation. Because they feel stressed most of the time, they are psychologically unprepared for the fact that relaxation can become a norm in life rather than an aberration. It is even more difficult for people to realize that the more relaxed they are, the more energy, stamina, awareness, clarity and strength they will have.

Energetic fitness enables the progressive release of tension and anxiety so that it becomes a living reality. It involves tuning in to your body and letting go of all your physical, emotional, mental, karmic, psychic and spiritual tension. Letting go means releasing chi blockages. Ultimately it means relaxing the nervous system so chi can strongly flow. Relaxation allows love, happiness and compassion to flourish.

## Myth #9:  Nonmovement exercises will not make you fit.

## Fact:  Breathing, standing and meditating are some of the most effective health and fitness practices you can adopt.

When I trained in karate, judo and jujitsu, I spent almost ten years vigorously learning to punch, throw and kick. I can remember my complete surprise during early phases of internal martial arts training in China when several masters said that the most effective exercise I could do for strength, speed and stamina was to stand. They all agreed that standing practice would enable me to get in touch with what was not relaxed in my body so I could release it. The basics for learning to stand will be introduced in the Chi Rev Workout in the last section of this book.

During my training as a chi gung healer in China, I learned that one of the most effective methods for improving the health of my patients was to teach them breathing practices, discussed in detail in Chapter 16. In later stages of my training in China, I learned that in order to become a superior martial artist, I had to practice Taoist meditation to release my deepest and most terrifying inner fears, angers, aggression and sadness. Not only did these methods make me strong and relaxed, they made it possible for me to recover from a devastating form of hepatitis and the car accident that injured my back. Over time I became incredibly healthy. The same chi practices have helped millions of people get fit, healthy and relaxed, and recover the sense of spontaneity and joy they had as children. They can do the same for you.

## Myth #10: I already know how to breathe; after all, I'm not dead!

## Fact: Most people do not breathe well.

According to medical and health associations, ninety percent of people are shallow breathers and forty percent use less than the full capacity of their lungs. As shallow breathers age, their lungs become weaker and they may experience shortness of breath, a precursor to ill health, weakness and depression. Although most people notice when they eat or sleep poorly, relatively few pay attention to their breathing. They are not aware that when they become angry or highly focused on their work, they hold their breath. Lack of oxygen to the brain revs up their nervous systems, making them tense and stressed. Learning the simple breathing exercises that are part of the Chi Rev Workout will help you discover your breathing patterns and help you change and improve them. If you only learn one lesson from this book, let it be that breath awareness is paramount to your health and longevity.

## Myth #11: Breathing is primarily about oxygenating the body.

## Fact: Breathing is primarily about getting the nervous system to relax while gently massaging the internal organs.

Breathing helps unravel the deadening effects of tension and anxiety. Every time we clutch, get uptight or have an adrenaline rush, stress locks into the nervous system and over time becomes habitual. As this happens, tension and constriction occur in the tissues, muscles, ligaments and tendons, cutting off some of the available oxygen and flow of blood in your body, particularly in your internal organs.

Longevity Breathing practices train you to focus on the negative breathing patterns you have and reverse them. They train you to calm down and relax. As you breathe fully and strongly, your internal organs get a gentle massage, which improves the circulation of fluids in and around them and makes them healthier. And, last but not least, you will also oxygenate your body more efficiently twenty-four hours a day. Focused, relaxed breathing is fundamental to all meditation practices.

## Myth #12: You have to have a special gift to feel chi.

## Fact: Anyone can learn to feel chi.

Chi is not some mysterious process that is only available to a rare few. In China, you can see small children holding and playing with imaginary balls. They are being trained to feel chi. However, many people in China as well as the West cannot feel the insides of their bodies. They do not understand the relationship between the body and mind, and they certainly have not been trained to feel chi.

Not only can chi practices help you feel your chi, but also they can help you recognize where it is blocked, as well as how to free, activate and strengthen it. Chi practices are not just about visualizing

your chi mentally. They help you develop your physical sensitivity
to how chi actually flows inside your body so eventually you will
become strong, feel well and eliminate your tension and anxieties.

## FROM HABITUAL TO RHYTHMIC

Maybe you have been frustrated with many of the health and fitness
programs you have tried and you agree with many of the facts
presented in this chapter. Myths have a great deal of power. That's
why advertising is so effective at making us spend money on stuff
that we probably don't need, that may not be good for us and often
doesn't deliver what is promised.

The challenge of the Chi Revolution is not just persuading you to
try these chi practices for yourself, but inspiring you to stick with
them and integrate them into your daily rhythm. Otherwise they
become just another "tasting" of the cornucopia of health and
exercise systems out there. Knowing something is good for you is
not the same as changing your habits to make them congruent
with that knowledge. We are addicted to our habits, many of them
conditioned and constantly reinforced by marketing mythology.

Activating and balancing chi has improved the health and wellness
of tens of millions of people. They understand that energetic fitness
affects their health as much as their diet, sleep habits and level of
physical activity. You can become energetically fit too. All it takes is
a little practice.

# Energetic Fitness: A New Paradigm for Longevity

One of my long-time students is a woman who began dancing professionally in her late teens. Sadly, she had to give up her career a few years later because of chronic and painful knee problems. She also suffered from abdominal difficulties from the aftermath of major surgery at age fifteen and years of eating disorders. Unfortunately, these kinds of complications are common for many dancers as well as other athletes. She tried many therapies, including the Alexander Technique, Rolfing and chiropractic work. Though they were somewhat helpful, she was no longer able to pursue a full-time dance career.

The abandonment of a childhood dream, the pressure to find a new path in life and the pain from her injuries left her with constant tension and worry. Finally she turned to tai chi and chi gung, primarily for stress reduction. She also had the desire to study something that offered the potential of a physical practice that could challenge her well into old age.

As she did her chi practices, she noticed a miracle happening. Not only did she become more relaxed, she also experienced a dramatic healing spreading throughout her whole body. To her surprise, one night in class she had the revelation that for the first time in over ten years she could feel what it was like to be hungry, a sensation she had lost during her teenage struggle with eating disorders.

As she adopted new body mechanics, she could acutely feel what old postural habits had done inside her body. Her joints began to mend because she no longer put them into jeopardy. She could fully train and bear her weight comfortably without the constant cloud of pain and discomfort.

At the age of thirty-seven, she is back to performing at a level of physical challenge she had not reached prior to her injuries. Her choreographer was stunned not only because her comeback occurred at an age when many dancers have to retire, but also because she became a better dancer than she was nearly a decade earlier.

As any professional athlete can tell you, this is almost unheard of. So what exactly did this woman tap into?

She used the healing power of her life-force energy; she has made her chi become abundant and strong. As the chi blockages progressively cleared, her body and mind healed. She has become energetically fit.

## A New Fitness Paradigm

Many Westerners associate fitness with exercises that get your heart rate up and your muscles strong. Yet the problems we have in today's modern world are not due to weak muscles or the inability to run for long distances. They develop because our nerves become shattered from the increasing speed and pace of life.

The Chi Revolution challenges you to take a step toward a different kind of fitness. It measures fitness by how much chi you have in your body and whether it is flowing smoothly or is blocked. I call it energetic fitness because when your chi runs like a strong river inside you, without blockages, you become incredibly fit and healthy. The key to energetic fitness is relaxing your nervous system while *simultaneously* supercharging your chi. The more relaxed you are during any activity, including any form of vigorous exercise, the more you enhance the circulation of chi and the stronger you become. Almost all of us are born with the innate ability to feel energy. At the end of a long workday, when you are stressed or sick, you probably feel the tangible depletion of your body's chi levels. When you feel good, or feel your body recharged after a good night's sleep, you feel energized.

*The smooth, balanced flow of chi—your life-force energy—is the single most important determinant to your health, vitality and happiness.* This concept, which is germane to Chinese medicine, is the primary reason why tai chi has been China's national health exercise for decades and is unlike any other sport or fitness craze.

## THE STRENGTH OF ENERGETIC FITNESS

Energetic fitness helps you access your inner ecology and feel inside your body. This in turn allows you to discover where chi is not running smoothly or where it might be stuck. There are three measures for how well chi flows in your body:

- The degree that chi can flow freely in your system;
- The quantity of chi you can store;
- The vibrational direction of your chi, toward the negative or positive.

By feeling your pulses, acupuncturists determine where chi is blocked and not flowing. Chi practices metaphorically give you the ability to take your own chi pulse. These practices teach you to recognize and progressively release the chi that is blocked in all your energy bodies as discussed in Chapter 3. When you begin to focus inside your body, you develop a succinct clarity about the quality of the energy that flows in your body rather than an abstract, ambiguous idea of it. Chi becomes a strong inner pulse that lets you know what is good for you personally and what is not, that is, whether you are moving toward life or death.

You will be able to measure your energetic fitness by how good you start feeling for longer periods during your day, not just after you exercise. At first, you might notice that you handle stress a little more easily; some of the aches and pains might fade away; you seem capable of concentrating without being distracted. At the end of the day, you might say something like, "I still have some energy left." As your chi gets progressively stronger, you begin replenishing your "chi account" at a faster rate than you are depleting it. You begin to store chi. In effect, you develop a chi reserve for when you need it, just like you have a savings account for unexpected expenses. Your creativity begins to wake up, along with your vitality and mental stamina. Chi practices free and strengthen your chi incrementally, in the same way water trickling over a rock first generates a small impression that can eventually turn into a magnificent canyon.

## ELIXIR FOR LIFE

You did not get sick or stressed in a day. Expecting to get well by taking some instant elixir meant for longevity and happiness is the lure of advertising. Like the buildup of pollutants in a river, chi blockages have collected inside you over many years. Over time and by consistently practicing some type of chi exercise, the pollutants will dissipate. Your internal rivers then run clean and freely.

You can begin with the simple breathing, scanning and movement exercises of the Chi Rev Workout found in the last section of this book. You could liken them to the notes and simple chords you learn when first taking piano or guitar lessons–you get the basics to build a foundation. The purpose is to orient you to focus inward and to begin recognizing some of your stagnant and trapped chi. Then you can choose among a variety of more complex practices, such as tai chi, chi gung, internal martial arts and TAO yoga, covered in more detail in the following chapters. These give you more interesting and satisfying chords and rhythms to work with. They activate your chi faster and teach you effective methods for releasing chi blockages and strengthening the flow of chi.

The more stuck energy you release, the more relaxed you feel, the more vitality you have and the healthier you become. It's a synergistic, holistic process. You have reversed the process of running yourself down to becoming healthier and moving toward life instead of death.

## SEPARATE AND COMBINE

All chi practices are not just about physical movements; they are effective methods developed over millennia to progressively give you access to your inner ecology and help you strengthen it. Ultimately, integration is the most central aspect of energetic fitness. A summary of this principle, "first separate, then combine," comes from the *Tai Chi Classics,* the authoritative source of tai chi principles for all the traditional styles, including the Yang, Wu and Chen. It is based on ancient Taoist texts and modern Chinese medical principles. First, you become aware of something that is independent of everything inside of you—separate from the system. Next, you combine it with the rest of you, the totality of everything else for which you are aware. Along that path, there are millions of little minicombinations and miniseparations before true integration of mind-body-spirit becomes a reality and increasingly more apparent inside you.

## NEI GUNG: THE SOPHISTICATED SCIENCE OF ENERGY FLOWS

Chi practices teach you that every external movement has both inner forms and outer forms. Your outer, external form is how your torso, head, arms and legs move through space. Your inner form is what you are doing inside your body with your mind, organs, fluids, nerves and energy. Developing awareness in every single body part inside you, both large and small, and understanding how they connect with each other are also parts of the inner form.

The Taoists call the science of how you develop strong energy flow or internal power *nei gung*.[1] Nei gung has sixteen components:

1. Breathing methods, from the simple to the more complex.
2. Feeling, moving, transforming, transmuting and connecting energy channels of the body.
3. Precise body alignments to prevent the flow of chi from being blocked or dissipated.
4. Dissolving blockages of the physical, emotional and spiritual aspects of ourselves.
5. Moving energy through the acupuncture meridians and other secondary channels of the body, including the energy gates.
6. Bending and stretching the body, both from the inside out and from the outside in.
7. Opening and closing (pulsing) all parts of the body's anatomy including the joints, soft tissues, fluids, internal organs, spine and brain as well as all the body's subtle energy anatomy.
8. Manipulating the energy of the external aura outside the body.
9. Making circles and spirals of energy inside the body, controlling the spiraling energy currents of the body and moving chi in the body at will.
10. Absorbing energy into and projecting energy away from any part of the body.
11. Controlling all the energies of the spine.
12. Controlling the left and right energy channels of the body.
13. Controlling the central energy channel of the body.
14. Learning to develop the capabilities and all uses of the body's lower tantien.
15. Learning to develop the capabilities and uses of the body's upper and middle tantiens.
16. Connecting every part of the physical and other energetic bodies into one, unified energy.

---

[1] Nei gung is discussed in more detail in the author's books, *Opening the Energy Gates of Your Body* and *The Power of Internal Martial Arts and Chi*, both published by Blue Snake Books.

The Chi Rev Workout in this book introduces some of the components of nei gung. Doing these powerful exercises will retrain your breathing patterns and biomechanical alignments as well as activate the energy of your aura. It will also teach you how to recognize blockages and how to absorb and project energy away from your body. Several energy-exercise systems are discussed in the next section to help you further develop and incorporate more aspects of your potential internal power.

## SPIRITUAL FITNESS

If you want to develop the spiritual side of yourself, the Taoists consider that energetic fitness is paramount in providing the necessary foundation. They point out that you don't construct a building from the top down; you start at the ground and work your way up.

First you must become healthy and have a stable, coherent mind and emotions. Then you are ready to advance to deeper aspects, or spiritual fitness through Taoist meditation. Before you can get to the core of your soul, you need to have cleared away enough blockages in your physical, emotional and mental bodies. This is the key to having strong and balanced chi running through your system. If you embark on a spiritual path before this, you can get stuck in some mental or emotional processes that can unravel and confuse your energy system for a long time. You could end up metaphorically spending thousands of hours trying to mentally process an energetic jumble running amok inside you. Frankly speaking, in most cases, you could do the appropriate energy exercises for a hundred hours and save yourself a lot of wasted time and unnecessary grief.

The purpose of Taoist meditation is to take you into your psychic, karmic and spiritual worlds. At this stage, you find that chi does not just run through you, it also runs through the entire physical and nonphysical universe, seeking connection, integration and balance. Energetic fitness helps you withstand the rigors of what you may find in these realms, which will be discussed in detail in Chapter 12.

# RELAXING INTO ENERGETIC FITNESS

As you progressively awaken the chi inside yourself, you develop the ability to use chi in your daily life to open up your human potential. Having copious reservoirs of chi propels you to higher performance on physical, emotional and mental levels. Your coordination, vitality, mental stamina, emotional stability and creativity can exceed that of most people. You become able to do things that the average person can't do—much like a super athlete.

I often get a kick out of asking one of the smallest older women at one of my classes to help me with a demonstration. I ask her to lie down with her knees bent and feet up in the air while leveraging around eight of the 200-plus-pound men against her feet. Each man adds his weight one by one, with the first man facing her and resting his stomach against her feet. Either I or one of my senior instructors makes tiny adjustments to maintain her alignments. She effortlessly pumps the men—weighing over 1,000 pounds—up and down without strain. Although it is beyond the woman's initial untrained ability, practicing will eventually allow her to do the exercise without any assistance from me or my instructors. People think it is magic when it is really just about proper alignments and the flow of chi.

As your chi becomes increasingly abundant, it fosters a "success breeds success" cycle that fills you with energy, relaxation and vitality. The plateaus you reach don't have an end; they progressively take you to one after another. And that is the real lure of these practices: they can engage you for life. Equally, they give you energy for life. Becoming energetically fit will supercharge your chi and relax your nerves.

Maybe you don't believe that having a seemingly illimitable abundance of energy is possible without pushing, creating tension and activating an adrenaline rush. See for yourself that the more you relax, the more energy and stamina you will have. If you practice, you don't have to take my word for it.

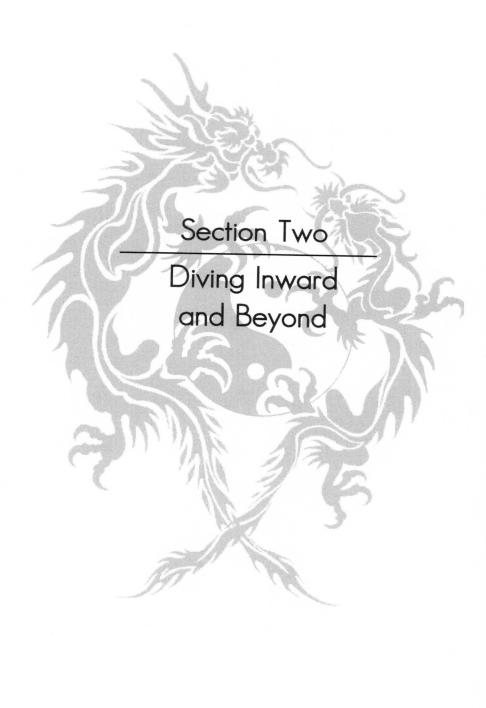

# Section Two

## Diving Inward and Beyond

# CHAPTER 8

# The Chi in Tai Chi and Chi Gung

Tai chi and chi gung (alternatively spelled *qigong* and *chi kung*) are among the most inspiring and popular chi practices to emerge out of China, with tens of millions of practitioners worldwide. These powerful self-healing exercises comprise the most sophisticated energetic-healing system ever devised. They can keep you energetically fit and healthy, and reduce anxiety and tension well into your old age. Chi cultivation was an essential part of the practices of ancient Taoist meditation adepts and is the foundation of chi gung, traditional Chinese medicine, acupuncture, tai chi and chi gung bodywork (chi gung tui na).

## GETTING STARTED WITH CHI GUNG

Chi gung literally means "energy work," from which hundreds of movement forms called sets have spawned. Some have origins in Taoism, others in Buddhism and martial arts. Although chi gung forms have different purposes, all focus on the various aspects of moving, cultivating and balancing chi. Medical chi gung exercises, a specific branch of Chinese medicine, boost the overall health of your body. They can also target specific ailments, such as arthritis, cancer, carpal tunnel syndrome, back pain, chronic fatigue and just about any type of dysfunction in the body.

The vast majority of China's medical chi gung exercises are based on activating the chi in the acupuncture pathways. Three such energy exercises are included in the Chi Rev Workout to help you balance and release stuck chi, and open up the flow of chi to your heart. These three exercises are part of a larger chi gung set, Dragon and Tiger, which will be discussed in detail in Chapter 15. Dragon and Tiger was specifically designed 1,500 years ago to abundantly and powerfully increase chi flow for incredible health benefits.

Although movements have a great deal to do with helping free up and mobilize your chi, your intent is equally powerful. The ancient Taoist saying is, "Chi follows your intent." The similar phrase in the West is "mind over matter." Today, cutting-edge research in science demonstrates that strong, positive intent can exert a powerful healing effect on yourself and others. According to renowned cellular biologist, Dr. Bruce Lipton, energetic messages that originate from our positive and negative thoughts profoundly affect healing processes at the level of the DNA in the cells.[1]

## TAI CHI: CHINA'S NATIONAL HEALTH EXERCISE

Chi gung's most well-known child in the West is tai chi, with over 200 million practitioners worldwide. Although many people may associate tai chi with martial arts, the majority of its practitioners use it purely as a potent health and longevity art. Of all medical exercises practiced in China, tai chi has been the predominant national health exercise over fifty years. Few health exercises have stood the test of time for as long as tai chi.

There are five major styles of tai chi[2]—Yang, Wu, Chen, Hao

---

[1] *The Biology of Belief: Unleashing the Power of Consciousness, Matter and Miracles* by Bruce H. Lipton (Mountain of Love Productions and Elite Press, 2005).

[2] See the author's book, *Tai Chi: Health for Life; How and Why It Works for Health, Stress Relief and Longevity* (Blue Snake Books, 2006) for comprehensive coverage of tai chi including practice guidelines for beginners and a review of forms.

and combination forms. Each takes a different approach to the movements commonly referred to as "forms," which include many variations or schools. Forms contain a number of repeated movements or postures that collectively comprise what is known as a "set." Some sets are short, containing fourteen to forty movements, and most can be performed in less than twenty minutes. Others are longer, some with as many as 128 movements, and could take up to an hour to practice.

Although numerous Westernized and nontraditional tai chi forms have been developed in recent years, many are extremely simplified. Little attention is paid to the precise body alignments and the energy mechanics that are critical to traditional tai chi. Studies show that even the simplified versions of tai chi still provide many health benefits. However, when tai chi incorporates correct body alignments and techniques for moving and cultivating chi, the benefits are vastly amplified and considerably more profound.

Having personally taught many thousands of students tai chi worldwide, I have found that most beginners are much better served by starting with traditional short forms because they require less commitment in terms of learning and practice. The short forms can give you most of the wide-ranging health benefits. You can later opt to learn the more complicated long forms, which offer all of tai chi's potential benefits, once you have established a base of knowledge and a solid practice rhythm.

## FINE-TUNING THE BODY FOR OPTIMAL HEALTH

The primary goals of tai chi and chi gung are to relax and regulate the central nervous system, to release physical and emotional stress and to promote mental and emotional well-being. These arts activate and strengthen the movement of chi throughout your body, which fine-tunes the body in three powerful ways:

○ Activating your nerves, making them stronger and less prone to stress.

○ Increasing the current of all the fluids moving in your body.
○ Causing a significant series of internal compressions and releases.

The movements of tai chi and chi gung precisely stimulate chi and systematically aid smooth and circular chi flow. As your body becomes balanced, the nerves release tension, resulting in a calming effect. Over time, as you continue your practice, you develop strength and resiliency; the body reconditions itself to counter stressful events with the relaxation response. You become trained to recognize when some place in your body tenses up or begins to be stressed so you can immediately stop yourself from going into the fight-or-flight response.

Increasing blood flow makes more oxygen available in the system, improving circulation and lowering blood pressure. Intrinsic to rejuvenation of every cell in your body is oxygen. As you oxygenate your cells, you become physically stronger and feel less depleted. Likewise, chi flow activates the fluids moving inside your joints. The result is greater flexibility, which is vitally important as we age. Stiff and stuck joints lead to dysfunction and, in serious cases, immobilization, considerably degrading the quality of life for many seniors. However, in this computer era, even school-age children experience tight necks, shoulders, backs and wrists. Many of the executives I teach report that tai chi and chi gung have dramatically reduced and even cured their carpal tunnel syndrome.

The movements of tai chi and chi gung also pump up your lymph flow, critical to the vitality and proper functioning of your immune system. They activate and smooth the flow of fluids up and down your spine and around your brain, which improves the general resiliency of your nervous system. Delivering nutrients and purging waste products depend entirely on the smooth-flowing current of your fluids. In this manner, every biological function in your body is upgraded. As you move and breathe, the inside of your body is constantly squeezed and released, closing and opening. Unlike normal exercise, contracting as well as relaxing your muscles is not part of the goal. Your muscles should remain relaxed throughout the entire exercise. In the case of neck, shoulder and all joint pain, the movement of fluids in the joints *and* the pressure of the fluids flowing in those joints both contribute to the release of tension and greater flexibility. Likewise, the series of compressions and releases inside your body serves as a very gentle, relaxing internal massage. This creates optimal health for your internal organs.

I ask my students if they would rather lose an arm or their liver. When the student is smart, he or she chooses an arm. Your internal organs are much more critical to the state of your health than external muscles or even the entire arm for that matter. So practicing tai chi or chi gung is no minor benefit to your overall health because these arts help keep your internal organs functioning at optimum capacity. Spending even a portion of the time you might spend at the gym to build up your muscles for an external appearance could be used to make you healthy from deep within. That glow you sometimes see people exude is not all about being physically fit. Some of the most physically fit people are also some of the unhealthiest people because well-being is not just about the way we look.

## BUILD ON EASY SUCCESSES

Tai chi and chi gung provide easy ways for you to directly experience putting your mind consciously inside your body. They progressively and systematically increase your internal body awareness. In the beginning, you tune into physical movements and sequences: basic body alignments, moderation, coordination, balancing, rudiments of Longevity Breathing and ways to bend and turn that will protect and lubricate your joints. As you practice, you begin to notice small effects growing into larger ones. Perhaps your arthritic fingers won't hurt all the time; maybe your headaches will be fewer and less severe. Perhaps your thoughts and emotions stop taking you on wild rollercoaster rides. Your practice is now taking hold inside you.

Intermediate and advanced practices help you directly feel and manage the flow of energy in your body, mind and spirit, via the system called nei gung, introduced in Chapter 7 (see p. 63). Nei gung is the Taoist science of how energy flows in humans. It has been codified and reduced to sixteen components—the roots from which every major chi gung system in China drew some or all of its original inspirations and techniques. Nei gung practices enable you to become increasingly aware of how your thoughts and emotions affect the flow of chi, both positively and negatively, and how to release chi blockages and manage the flow of your energy.

Nei gung is an essential part of all high-level Taoist tai chi, chi gung, internal martial arts, yoga, sexual practices and meditation. Learning and incorporating aspects of nei gung is what makes tai chi, chi gung and other chi practices ever-evolving arts—ones that will engage, interest and inspire you throughout your life. The more you practice, the more effective they become.

## Low Impact Is High Performance

Tai chi and chi gung are primarily low-impact exercises that can be safely practiced by people of all age groups and body types, including the overweight. Some forms of chi gung can be safely practiced while recovering from surgery or severe illness since many exercises can be done while sitting or lying down.

The term "low impact" is a misnomer since these exercises have a significant impact on the body. It refers to the fact that they are gentle on the joints, that they are done slowly, in contrast to aerobics, and that they do not jack up the heart rate. Low impact also refers to the importance of following the principles of the seventy percent rule which greatly helps reduce anxiety and fine-tune the body faster than going for the push of high-impact exercises. The message is this: Keeping it low impact as you practice gives you high-octane performance.

# Skill Is Born from Practice

Given the significant benefits of tai chi and chi gung, why have so few Westerners taken up chi practices? Some of the reasons have a great deal to do with the myths about health and fitness many of us have adopted. Others have to do with resistance to going inside and dealing with our internal miseries. Another reason is that many people find that the movements are not easy to learn. Even some professional athletes and dancers can initially find that they are challenged by the coordination involved. For example, some get frustrated because they cannot make the left hand move at the same speed as their right foot, or remember which direction to turn, or which hand or foot to move forward.

Be patient with yourself. It takes most people anywhere from a few days to a few weeks or more to comfortably assimilate any set of new physical movements or energetic principles. It also takes time for the body to relax and soften enough to become conscious of and to be able to accommodate the more complex physical and energetic dynamics. The important thing to remember as you start practicing is that you don't have to be an expert to benefit from tai chi or chi gung. Even done poorly, these arts can provide health benefits. As you gain experience and the ability to adhere to body alignments and energy mechanics, you'll find that the quality of your movements improves dramatically as well as your overall health. Developing patience is inherent to any new skill, and tai chi and chi gung are particularly helpful for cultivating fortitude.

# Western Medical Studies Confirm What the Chinese Have Known for Centuries

Practitioners of tai chi and chi gung tell many inspirational stories of how they have been cured of high blood pressure, carpal tunnel syndrome, polio, chronic fatigue, arthritis and hepatitis. My students frequently tell me how they have recuperated from illness or surgery at record speeds, how much their stress and anxiety decreases, how they don't often come down with colds or flu and many other amazing personal accounts.

Their stories are now being confirmed by Western medical studies. Formal studies help healers in Western traditional and alternative communities become comfortable recommending tai chi and chi gung to their patients. Three studies have confirmed that tai chi and chi gung boost the immune system, mitigate arthritis and lower blood pressure. This demonstrates some of the powerful effects of these ancient healing systems.

## Boosting Immunity

A study by the University of California, Los Angeles, found that those who practiced tai chi for forty-five minutes a day experienced up to a fifty percent increase in their memory T cells, which boost immunity to many diseases including simple colds, shingles and cancer.[1] The study also found that tai chi helps reduce the fear and anxiety that accompanies cancer and mitigates the effects of chemotherapy and radiation. Over the years, I've worked with many students who have had the unfortunate experience of being diagnosed with cancer. Remarkably, many have maintained their quality of life and some have even healed themselves to the point of astonishing their doctors with total remission.

## Alleviating Arthritis

Arthritis limits the activity of over seven million Americans and is second only to heart disease as a cause of work disability. Arthritis is expected to increase dramatically as the baby boomers age. By 2020, an estimated 60 million Americans, or almost twenty percent of the population, will be affected by arthritis. Two major studies where two different styles of tai chi were practiced confirm that tai

---

[1] Irwin MR, Pike JL, Cole JC, and Oxman MN. 2003. "Effects of a Behavioral Intervention, Tai Chi Chih, on Varicella-Zoster Virus Specific Immunity and Health Functioning in Older Adults" in *Psychosomatic Medicine* 65: 824-830.

chi alleviates arthritis pain. Tufts-New England Medical Center studied rheumatoid arthritis sufferers with an average age of fifty.[1] After three months of doing Yang style tai chi twice a week, they had fewer tender joints than a similar study group that simply did stretching exercises. In Australia, three Korean professors and Dr. Paul Lam, a family physician, in collaboration with two universities, conducted a randomized study of seventy-two adults with arthritis.[2] After three months of practicing Sun style tai chi, patients had thirty-five percent less pain, twenty-nine percent less stiffness, twenty-nine percent more ability to perform daily tasks such as climbing stairs, improved abdominal muscles and better balance. The study was widely publicized by the Arthritis Foundation of Australia, which now officially recommends tai chi as an effective alternative therapy.

*I had a sports injury to my right thumb many years ago. It had become arthritic to a point that I could not touch it or pull my keys from my pocket without extreme pain. Chi gung got me my thumb back without surgery.*

*As an architect I needed that thumb to draw! So, one day, sitting at my desk, I thought of pulsing the joint, breathing energy in and out, something I learned from one of my nei gung classes with Bruce Frantzis. After about five minutes, the joint started to pulsate with a force, something that felt like an electromagnetic field, and energy started moving out the end of my thumb. It felt like electricity. To my surprise, the pain went away. This was about ten years ago. The joint is now pain free even though it still looks damaged. If I ever feel a twinge of pain starting, I just pulse the joint to give it a tune up.*

—Bob Carter, Architect
Jackson, Wyoming

---

[1] Wang C, Roubenoff R, Lau J, Kalish R, Schmid CH, Tighiouart H, Rones R, and Hibberd PL. 2005. "Effect of Tai Chi in Adults with Rheumatoid Arthritis" in *Rheumatology* 44: 685-687.
[2] Song R, Lee EO, Lam P, and Bae SC, 2003. "Effects of Tai Chi Exercise on Pain, Balance, Muscle Strength and Perceived Difficulties in Physical Functioning in Older Women with Osteoarthritis: A Randomized, Clinical Trial" in *The Journal of Rheumatology,* Sep; 30(9): 2039-44.

## Healing Others with Chi

After you have healed yourself and made your chi very strong, you can develop your chi practices even further and share your life-force energy to help heal others.

Chi gung tui na is a special branch of Chinese medicine that is designed to unblock, free and balance chi in others. Instead of using needles, as acupuncturists do, you learn to project your energy into your patients with and without hands-on techniques. In order to heal others with chi, you must first learn to unlock and free your own chi and control the specific pathways through which chi flows. You need to be able to feel your chi strongly so that you know how to identify strength and weaknesses in chi flow in others. Finally, you need to learn to project chi to help your patients heal from illness and blockages. Core chi practices will serve as a foundation.

Part of chi gung tui na training is learning how to keep from becoming physically, spiritually or emotionally exhausted. This practice has several important components:

- Protecting yourself from absorbing the energy of your patients.
- Regenerating your own energy after putting out chi on behalf of others.
- Cultivating compassion for your patients.
- Doing regenerative practices. The rule of thumb is that, to avoid burnout, you should spend up to a quarter of the time you spent working on patients doing regenerative practices on yourself.

## Lowering Blood Pressure

According to recent estimates, nearly one in three American adults has high blood pressure. It is often called the "silent killer" because when uncontrolled, high blood pressure can lead to stroke, heart attack, heart failure or kidney failure. A study of sixty-two sedentary seniors who did both tai chi and light aerobics was conducted by the Johns Hopkins School of Medicine.[1] Results showed that tai chi's gentle movements were as effective in significantly lowering blood pressure as aerobic exercise. Although the study found that both types of exercise were equally effective, researchers concluded that tai chi had an edge for seniors because it is a low-impact, light-intensity activity. Tai chi can be performed anytime, anywhere, and requires no change of shoes or special clothing. This is especially helpful for elders who might have limited budgets or who identify exercise with strenuous activity.

*After studying chi gung and Wu style tai chi with Bruce Frantzis for a year, my at-rest heart rate dropped from an average of about 60–65 bpm to about 50–52 bpm, and blood pressure readings dropped about eight to ten points on both the systolic and diastolic ranges. I am more than thankful to have these practices available to assist in maintaining my general good health.*

—Daniel Weismann, Graphic Artist
Albuquerque, New Mexico

# FINDING TEACHERS

Most cities and towns in America, Canada and Europe offer classes in tai chi and chi gung. Teachers vary in their degree of competence, both in their ability to be proficient in the movements and in their ability to communicate what's important, verbally and non-verbally. Although China has a long-established hierarchy of teacher competence, Western countries have no equivalent. There are no recognized rating and accreditation systems, no uniforms or colored belts and no standardized method for grading competence.

---

[1] Young DR, Appel LJ, and Jee SH. 1999. "T'ai Chi Lowers Blood Pressure" in *Journal of the American Geriatrics Society* 47: 277-284.

Only a few teachers offer formal instructor trainings, such as those that I offer.

Teachers also vary in their focus. Some focus on health and stress reduction, others on martial arts or meditative aspects. Some have a method of teaching important fundamentals and, more rarely, aspects of nei gung. The core chi gung programs my instructors and I teach were deliberately chosen because they are among the oldest, most effective and most treasured of Taoist energy practices.[1] They are ideal for progressively incorporating the major components of nei gung, as discussed in Chapter 7, in a manner that Westerners understand. They provide students with the foundations necessary for clearly and systematically learning and advancing their chi practices.

Good teachers can positively influence you and possibly change your life for the better. Incompetent ones can turn you off forever. If you are in city that offers you a choice, take the time to survey teachers to find the one who is right for you. It can make all the difference in how quickly you advance and integrate the principles of tai chi and chi gung into your daily activities. I encourage you to begin a tai chi and/or chi gung practice and possibly even learn how to teach it to help others. There will be a great need for competent teachers in the years to come.

---

[1] To learn more about chi gung and the sixteen-part nei gung system, visit EnergyArts.com.

# The Secret Power of Internal Martial Arts

The art of all internal martial arts—ba gua, tai chi and hsing-i—is to fight with total relaxation, balanced emotions and no muscular tension. As with all chi practices, internal martial arts train you to be extremely healthy, relaxed and focused, in body, mind and spirit.

The word "internal" is used because the movement of chi in the body and your intent give you the power to supercharge your physical movements. Developing speed, strength and stamina in the internal martial arts is about developing chi, not muscular strength. Focusing on muscular force will impede your ability to feel and move chi through the body. Fighting in the external martial arts, such as karate and tae kwon do, is often accompanied by screaming, yelling, tensing and the making of animal-like contortions. The purpose is to help practitioners focus their power and frighten their opponents. These emotional rushes release adrenaline and other stress-related hormones, which may not only harm the body, but also eventually serve as a form of self-hypnosis. If a punch, kick or throw causes a scream to be constantly repeated, you can be sure it will also cause the body to tense inside. Fighting relaxed, without aggression, anger or adrenaline releases, makes for the most lethal fighters. Releasing adrenaline and other hormones inhibits the flow of chi, weakening the body and, by extension, decreasing the flow of chi power.

The question is this: How can one remain internally relaxed and calm in a combat situation? Whether you have an interest in the internal martial arts or in becoming any kind of fighter, the training methods serve as examples of the potentials of chi. Many of the lessons can be applied to daily living.

## Overcoming Aggression

In terms of stress, the chief issue in martial arts training is how to overcome an aggressive biology patterning that causes the mind and body to tense in fighting situations. A martial artist might have a strong punch, but the real test of his ability is if he throws the punch with uncontrolled anger or if he maintains a calmness of mind throughout. Is he addicted to the rush and power feelings that adrenaline gives him, or can he fight with a mind that is smooth even with chaos around him?

Calming the monkey mind becomes a major issue in the internal martial arts. On a pragmatic level, once you become tense, agitated or gripped with an emotion such as anger or fear, vulnerability presents itself. This weak point can therefore be exploited by your opponent. There is a gap. Maybe you hold your breath; maybe you hesitate; or maybe you have a moment of indecision about where or how to strike. Every place inside where you hold anger, fear, bad memories or some limitation of the mind is where a gap might emanate. When you have a gap, your mind, body and spirit will be incapable of functioning with a smooth, unified flow, and this inadequacy makes it possible for your opponent to defeat you.

One of my ba gua masters, Wang Shu Jin, would fool his opponents into thinking there was a gap by softening and completely relaxing his stomach. An opponent would unwittingly come in for a strike to

Wang's stomach, only to have his arm sucked in. Then Wang would fill his stomach with chi, expanding his muscles until they were like the skin of a drum and deflect the opponent backwards. Often times he would break the hand or dislocate the shoulder of his opponent in the process.

The optimal fighter will stay completely relaxed even when facing possible injury or death. He knows that only by doing so will he have the highest probability of not being hurt because when his chi is flowing, he will be stronger, faster and more present. The foundation skill for all internal martial arts is the same as with all chi practices: how to relax the nervous system so chi will flow strongly. All training is then to learn to maintain the chi flow in any situation. The purpose of sparring in internal martial arts is to flush out and confront any chi blockages such as fear, anger or mental confusion in a practice arena rather than the battlefield, where it could be a life or death situation.

## PRACTICE STANDING TO GET MORE CHI

While training in Japan, I asked one of my tai chi masters, Chang I Jung, if there was any one thing that I could practice that would lead to most strongly developing my internal power. He instructed me to stand, first in the most basic posture that is included in the Chi Rev Workout and later in other postures as well. Religiously following that advice, I trained myself to stand in various postures for two hours or more each day. After two years, I was able to surpass most of his advanced students—some of whom had over a decade experience practicing tai chi and other internal martial arts.

Why would repetitive standing allow me to achieve such dramatic feats? Standing taught me to unequivocally feel where my chi was moving or not moving, blocked or unblocked, smooth or not smooth. Most importantly, I learned how to release stuck chi and allow it to flow freely. The more relaxed I became, the more my chi began to powerfully flow inside me. As my chi began flowing freely, the more potent and faster I became as a martial artist. As my chi became smoother, my kicks and punches became stronger and more effective. Also, I gained a less glamorous skill—my mental agility became more developed.

## Using the Chi of Your Opponent

Internal martial arts are relationship arts—they require you to feel and connect to the chi of your opponent. To the extent that you can become conscious and sensitive to how your chi is interacting with that of your opponent, you will be an effective fighter. But you cannot even hope to tune into the chi of your opponent if you first are not tuned into the chi flowing within you.

The force of chi is like an exploding bullet that never really leaves the gun; the power never discharges, it circulates within. Martial artists first learn this sticking ability by touching and adhering to someone else's skin as they both move. Over time, this progresses to where they sensitively track the chi emitted by different parts of the body—sensing it without sight or tactile input. Then, when they fight, they look for where their opponent's chi is absent, weak or fluctuating. It could be something as gross as a locked joint or as subtle as a gap of consciousness, such as blanking out from an emotional blockage, if only for a microsecond.

## Intent Moves Chi

The way in which you get power in all the internal martial arts is by applying your intent to accomplish very specific procedures. Whether it is a technique for fighting, a form or a posture or a method for releasing blocked chi, your mind must ultimately mobilize your chi. Intent moves chi, chi moves blood and blood brings strength. So it follows that if precisely directed, the stronger your intent, the stronger the flow of chi. This important principle applies to all other chi practices as well. Science is now demonstrating how your intent exerts profound effects on yourself and others.[1]

## MASTERING NEI GUNG

Ultimately, the way to harness chi and intent and apply it to fighting movements is through feeling, developing, strengthening and moving chi. This involves mastery of the sixteen nei gung components—the heart of all chi practices—discussed in Chapter 7. Once chi really energizes the body, it functions optimally, so you can perform even the most precise movements. As chi grows, the unconscious and conscious mind unify with increasing force. Mind and energy dance with and reinforce each other. One does not exist independently of the other. Ultimately, nei gung is about developing a strong connection between body, mind and spirit continuously and circularly, without gaps. The phrase from the *Tai Chi Classics* sums up the goal of nei gung training: "From posture to posture the internal energy is unbroken." That is to say, chi is abundant and the person is wide awake in mind, body and spirit *without disconnection.*

The extraordinary sensitivity to chi provided by the nei gung system differentiates the internal from the external martial arts. The ability to clear chi in all the energy channels and to highly fuse the mind and chi is rarely, if ever, learned through karate, jujitsu, tae kwon do and other external martial arts. When your chi is like that of a strong waterfall, you have unity of body, mind and spirit—the true secret of internal martial arts.

## THE SPIRITUAL WARRIOR

At the very highest levels of internal martial arts training, martial artists can embark on the path of the spiritual warrior. In doing so, they must overcome and transcend their deepest inner enemies,

---

[1] Numerous studies are described in *The Intention Experiment: Using Your Thoughts to Change Your Life and the World* by Lynne McTaggart (Free Press, 2007).

the ones embedded in their psychic, karmic and spiritual energy bodies. They must conquer their deepest afflictive emotions and addictions. They must bring their internal senses to a high level of clarity. At the more advanced levels, internal martial arts training can be called the path of the spiritual warrior.[1] Tools for fighting are found in the body and in the mental strategies that accompany combat skills. Spirituality is found in the martial artist's heart, mind and spirit, the energies that allow the person to function and connect to others, directing that person's awareness and intention.

In the Taoist tradition, training in the spiritual martial arts integrates fighting techniques with Taoist meditation so that the spiritual warrior can:

o Develop relaxed, continuous and unbroken attention for long periods, without becoming tense, distracted or dissociated.
o Cut the roots of what allows inner demons to prevail.
o Become unattached to worldly or spiritual illusions.
o Integrate body, mind and spirit in all of his or her energy bodies.
o See into and liberate the core of his or her soul.

Instead of battling and defeating external opponents in the quest for spirituality, martial artists tackle the internal, spiritual foes that live in the depths of their souls. They take on the greatest challenge of human existence: to become relaxed, balanced, compassionate and free at the deepest core of themselves. If successful, they will emerge forever connected to—not separated or alienated from—all of life's experiences.

---

[1] See the author's book, *The Power of Internal Martial Arts and Chi*, Chapter 9, "The TAO of Spiritual Martial Arts."

# TAO Yoga and the Man in the Suitcase

W hen I was living in Tokyo at the age of nineteen, I studied Hatha yoga with Perr Wynter, a Norwegian man. His first teacher was an Indian yogi who lived up the fjord from him. When he was in his twenties, Perr went to India to study at the Shivananda Ashram and became an exceptional Hatha yogi. When he took some time to travel in Malaysia, his money and passport were stolen. So, in order to earn money, he worked for a circus and eventually became well known for folding himself into a suitcase. What was interesting was that Perr could do virtually any Hatha yoga posture that existed. He was the yoga teacher of Yamaguchi Gogen, the legendary founder of Goju Kai Karate Do.

Since we both also studied aikido and tai chi together, I came to understand that Perr's chi did not really flow. He had a kind of semispastic quality to his movements and he was known as a rather poor student of the martial arts even after years of practicing. Despite being extremely healthy and strong, he was relatively uncoordinated. How could this human rubber band not have energy flowing in his body? It wasn't until I trained in the internal martial arts, chi gung and static Taoist postures (which I refer to and teach as TAO yoga), all of which powerfully developed my own chi, that I was able to figure out Perr's perplexing situation. Perr had stretched his fibers to the extent that he became extremely flexible. He had precise mechanical control of his body, but he was not a relaxed person. He did not have the fluidity and ease that tai chi and aikido can give you. He was not relaxed in the sound of his voice or the way in which he moved.

The lesson I learned was that people can do yoga, be super stretched and flexible and yet still be incredibly tense with chi bound inside them. Perr's nerves were taut and so was the energy that ran through him.

## TAO YOGA: USE YOUR BREATH TO HELP YOU RELAX

The primary emphasis in TAO yoga is to stimulate the flow of chi and free any blocked chi. By combining gentle postures and Longevity Breathing derived from ancient Taoist techniques, the body's energy channels are progressively opened and the flow of chi is thereby activated and strengthened. TAO yoga has many gentle, seated postures, held from two to five minutes each. Because the postures require virtually no muscular effort, they enable you to "go internal" easily, to focus on feeling where the chi is blocked and to gently free it up. You quickly become aware of where chi is flowing and where it is not.

As you hold a posture or move to the next one, you are taught to breathe continuously and smoothly from the belly. The breath is never held or restricted; there is no forcing of the breath and no attempt to push or elongate the length of the inhale and exhale. Smooth, continuous breathing enables your nervous system to relax as you hold a posture or move to the next one. There is no activation of any physical, mental or emotional tension or contraction. Chi blockages therefore encounter progressively less resistance in the posture you are holding and are able to release until your chi eventually has a natural, free-flowing quality.

Conversely, holding the breath during postures, a common practice in many forms of Hatha yoga and its modern spinoffs, can reinforce stress patterns that many people have unconsciously adopted when they are fearful, angry or tense. This is probably what happened to Perr. Holding the breath with tension creates a tremendous amount of internal pressure, which rattle the nervous system and block the flow of chi in the body. It can also lead to out-of-control explosions of negative emotions.

The use of Longevity Breathing techniques—discussed in detail in Chapter 16—and TAO yoga's gentle, non-forcing postures, helps break the deeply conditioned association that links holding the breath with stressful events. Psychologists tell us there is no stopping a bad behavior, only replacing it with a new one. Habits of tension need to be broken and replaced with habits of relaxation. This is a primary goal of TAO yoga, Longevity Breathing and all chi practices for that matter.

Here, a major dictum of Taoism prevails: Tension, of whatever kind, inhibits relaxation and is difficult to maintain. Relaxation frees energy and gives you more stamina and strength. By redirecting your mind and breath to feel the flow of chi in a posture, you lose the sense of any need to push. In turn, your nervous system relaxes even more and opens up the possibilities of real transformation inside you.

## RELAXATION FOR EVERYONE

TAO yoga can be practiced by people of any age or body type. Because the emphasis is not on the stretch or on developing complex postures, there is no feeling of competition to "look good in the posture." Injuries are also a rare occurrence. Although many of the postures in TAO yoga resemble the beginning and intermediate postures of Hatha yoga, TAO yoga never forces your body or asks you to do extreme stretches. Instead of focusing on the external qualities of a given posture as in most forms of yoga, TAO yoga is meant to help you put your awareness into your body. There is little concern about how far you can lengthen tissue, muscles, ligaments and tendons. Rather, you put your attention on releasing chi blockages from within the body. Conversely, when your efforts are directed at holding difficult postures or on stretching the muscles, the nervous system reacts by closing up the energy channels. A negative feedback loop is created. Although you can force the muscles to stretch, your body can become incredibly tense and shut down. You will naturally begin to stretch further over time as you progressively relax without the strain and push.

## RELAX TO STRETCH

Most yoga practitioners stretch to relax. The Taoists take it from the other direction: They relax in order to stretch. I demonstrate this point in my classes by having one of my more flexible students do a full spilt. Next, I ask her to repeat the process of slowly going down into a spilt, only this time I instruct her to stop when she reaches any tension or contraction—anything that would indicate a chi blockage. Not surprising, she finds she might only be able to go down a few inches. Now she uses her breath and internal focus to relax the blockage and gets the chi to flow. She does not force her body to the point where any nerves clench whether at the site of the obstruction or any other place in her body. As her nervous system relaxes, the chi blockages encounter less and less resistance and eventually release. The student repeats this process, only moving downwards and going into a deeper split as each blockage she encounters is freed up.

Once you place your awareness on the smooth, balanced flow of energy in the body, the nervous system creates a natural link to the feeling of relaxation. A natural, positive feedback loop is created. The process does not take years or even months; it can happen in the first few TAO yoga sessions. However, as you practice, you'll become aware of ever-deeper layers that will help you let go of more subtle blockages. As one of my students told me during a TAO yoga workshop, "When I go into a posture, I find it easy to feel the relationship of my breath to my chi, and how they are affected by my thoughts and emotions. For this reason, I find that TAO yoga makes it dramatically easier for me to find and to let go of whatever binds me."

## A Natural Bridge to Meditation

The original intent of yoga was to achieve stillness in the body as the necessary foundation for meditation—not all the complicated gymnastics we see today. Yoga was primarily developed to help students maintain a comfortable sitting posture. In fact, the Sanskrit term *asana* literally means "seat"—the way in which your body rests on the ground when you meditate. Clearly, your body has to be stretched out to a certain degree or you will get some physical pain after sitting for a few hours. This is especially true after a few weeks or years of doing this every day as some yogis do on the path to spiritual enlightenment.

As you focus on the circularity of your breath and chi from one posture to another, it becomes easier to let go of your thoughts and emotions. You can locate blockages in your body and attend to them without all the internal dialogue that wants to fight or control them. The more you let go, the more you relax, the more smoothly your chi flows, the more open and present you become. It's a synergistic process that leads you to a point of stillness inside yourself.

TAO yoga is known as a bridge to TAO meditation because it is so effective at quickly calming the monkey mind. Many of my students who are new to chi practices have found it to be the easiest way for them to get a sense of their bodies, such as feeling their internal organs. The movements are slow and steady enough for them to maintain their concentration yet challenging enough to keep them from spacing out the way many of them do while learning breathing and other beginning energy practices. When they feel clear and present to their experiences, most find that they naturally reach a still point. And reaching a profound, relaxed stillness is the stable foundation necessary for allowing your spiritual path to unfold.

# The TAO of Sex

Making love is like cooking a three-course meal. Ideally, you want to make sure all the needed cooking utensils and ingredients are accounted for and working in the kitchen. Everything is present. First comes the appetizers, or foreplay, which can become a full meal of its own; next, the main course, or intercourse; and finally the dessert—physical satisfaction, release, relaxation and increased post-coital, emotional bonding. You can also choose to have spiritual dessert—sexual practices that lead you to internal balance, compassion and universal love. Each course has its pleasures and joys. But to fully discover and experience them, you have to get the chi fully going in yourself and your partner.

## TAOIST SEXUAL PRACTICES

As people make love, the chi in their bodies amplifies and swells pretty much on its own. We feel more alive, creative and vibrant as chi becomes more abundant and intensified. Our blood and other fluids flow more strongly, making us feel tingly and flushed. For many, the release that follows orgasm is often the time when we feel most relaxed and when the mental and negative emotional chatter seem to disappear. We feel fully present to our experience.

Now the Taoists are not concerned with much of the cultural, moral and religious baggage that sex might be associated with in the West. They are more interested in exploring energetic motivations and, as such, the Taoist practices were designed by studying consenting heterosexual adults using safety precautions and no force. All things considered, they approach sexuality unabashedly and pragmatically to explore the potential of stimulating free-flowing chi inside people. The Taoist sexual practices are categorized in two segments:

- *Sexual chi gung*—techniques that increase the sensitivity and awareness of chi flows within yourself and your partner, including techniques that help you achieve many of the healing benefits of any chi practice.
- *Sexual meditation*—methods that lead to profound religious experience often called the divine, enlightenment, emptiness and universal love.

## SEX MAKES IT EASY TO FEEL YOUR CHI

Feeling your chi is just plain easier during and after sex. Feeling your chi in one instance makes it easier to feel it in other contexts, such as by yourself while doing the Chi Rev Workout, tai chi or chi gung.

The sexual act itself causes your energy to naturally become obvious, vibrant and accessible to you. If you have a very difficult time feeling what's going on within your body or feeling your chi—and many do—the easiest time to make it possible to feel anything related to your life force is during the sexual act. This is because sex, which unleashes the procreative capacity, also unleashes extreme human creativity and awareness. When the inside of your body becomes high, hot and fully functioning, the capacity to become aware at physical, energetic, mental and psychic levels intrinsically opens up.

So the sexual act is a natural method for enhancing your ability to feel what was previously numb and unaware. Because your chi is so accessible to you, it becomes easier to learn and incorporate the sixteen components of nei gung into any other practice to feel, strengthen and gain control of your chi. Sex can be likened to a form of super chi gung that can awaken and charge your chi.

## RELAX INTO SEX

Many people, even physical laborers who work twelve-hour days, are able to have sex all night, especially when they are young. Although the body is tired, the nerves are not. Others, who might not have even expended much physical energy in their workday, have no sex at all because they are stressed out. Anxiety and tension do not make room for relaxation, and that includes sex. When the nerves are shot and depleted, which is common in our overwhelmed, overscheduled, overcaffeinated and technology-driven lives, our interest in sex and ability to have it diminishes. When the sex drive is shut down by the central nervous system, particularly those nerves that are stimulated during sexual activity, it makes people incapable of feeling and responding. This is especially true after long periods of excessive visual and mental stimulation with no physical outlet. It is the case for people who work on computers much of the day; they experience nervous rather than physical exhaustion. Men can't "get it up" when they are uptight because their nerves are shot and the blood does not flow into the sexual organs. It's the same for women who find themselves "dry": When people are anxious and stressed, the sexual fluids just do not flow.

Sexual chi practices help release the nerves and increase blood flow—without pills and salves. What does that mean? The more relaxed you become, the more easily the chi begins to flow; more abundant chi leads to a greater capacity for cultivating sexual vitality and pleasurable sex.

## DEEPLY CONNECT WITH YOURSELF

From the Taoist point of view, strengthening your chi and specifically directing its flows during sex helps you achieve all the wonderful benefits of any chi practice. When all that juice is flowing, you learn to guide your chi so it is not just some random supercharge. Feeling your chi during sex makes it easier to get out of your head and connect to yourself. Harnessing your chi can help release blockages, make you healthier and allow the positive emotions, such as happiness and compassion, to flourish. You become more open to your emotions and mental energies, so you can effectively smooth out the suppressed, uneven and jangled emotions. You can use that expansive sense of chi not just to stop the mental chatter but to increase mental capacities and bring out your creativity.

## PARTNER EXERCISES

For millennia, Taoists have found that one of the easiest ways to directly contact another person's consciousness is while making love. It takes dramatically more time, skill, power and finesse to directly contact another person's consciousness from a distance than it is during sex. There is an inherent connection in the act of making love.

As you release the blockages in yourself, you become less self-absorbed and more open and present to someone else. As you become more connected to yourself, it becomes increasingly easier to feel more deeply for someone else. And, in that space, a wonderful merging, you can sense the chi of the other person as much as you experience the chi in yourself. When chi flows strongly between you, it becomes a healing and smoothing force, especially important when you are sharing a life together and encountering the strains inherent to the human condition. You can take that vibrant, strong energy running between you, relax it and take the growing intimacy between you to much deeper levels.

# PRACTICING SEXUAL CHI GUNG

As with all chi practices, sexual chi gung techniques are meant to increase the sensitivity and awareness of chi flows within you and your partner. You go inside, become aware of raw sensations, allow them to strengthen your chi flow and get rid of blockages. The process of waking up and making the body conscious is about feeling, not thinking. Initial techniques help you become conscious of chi flow in your own body and then in your partner's body during intercourse. This inherently increases sexual pleasure between you and your partner—connecting and sharing.

These techniques can be fairly basic, such as finger exercises that you do by yourself to increase sensitivity to both yourself and your partner while ensuring that your fingers and hands don't cramp up after a few minutes of foreplay. Other practices help you and your partner relax during foreplay, intercourse and afterwards. Still other practices put both you and your partner to work to harness your chi to relax the nervous system, self-heal and allow the mental and emotional intimacy to flourish.

Sexual chi gung, although a longstanding tradition in Taoism, is seldom taught in the West. I have taught a few classes in Europe, where sexual mores are not as straight-laced as in America, yet find that even there, cultural and religious conditionings work against it.[1] You can realize many of the benefits of sexual chi gung by learning other practices that help you feel and strengthen your chi. The Chi Rev Workout is among those foundational practices, which also include tai chi and chi gung. At the very least, they will increase and help you maintain your sexual vitality and pleasure throughout your life.

---

[1] Some of the techniques of sexual chi gung are found in the author's book, *The Great Stillness* (North Atlantic Books, 2001).

## PRACTICING SEXUAL MEDITATION

All chi practices inherently contain methods to take you into the depths of your consciousness. The ancient and well-established tradition of Taoist sexual meditation was also passed down by Lao Tse and Chuang Tse. These practices give you the opportunity to discover deep intimacy that transcends flesh and personality. Sexual meditation can be a direct path to releasing the deepest blockages in yourself and your partner, including those at the psychic, karmic and spiritual levels, in order to develop the full flowering of the human soul. It can help you uncover the possibilities of spirit by working with the eight energetic and spiritual bodies discussed in Chapter 3 (see pp. 23-24). Finally, it can guide you toward a profound inner religious experience, often called the varying degrees of enlightenment, emptiness and universal love.

In China, sexual meditation methods were only shared with initiates and taught by masters, whereas sexual chi gung techniques could be taught to and shared with outsiders. Being given access to sacred meditation material was considered a great privilege and honor. It was not a right, not something to be bought and sold without any more responsibility attached than merely to be present when the information was taught. Genuine traditional Eastern meditation practices are not for everyone, especially those involved with deeply exploring human sexuality. Here you can lose the distinct boundaries between the bodies and minds of you and your lover as being two separate beings—boundaries that are at some primal bedrock of the ego's sense of psychological security and identity.

Equally, in prolonged, in-depth training, both participants can each go into completely uncharted psychic territories. Here any form of sexual morality based on the "should's," "could's," "must's" and "maybe's" of social or religious convention might become meaningless and disappear as you both move into the psychic realm and, ultimately, emptiness. Over time during sexual meditation, it is imperative that you become willing to completely open up and be naked in front of your partner both literally and metaphorically—not only in the obvious physical sense, but also on the emotional, mental, psychic and karmic levels. Your physical body is only a fairly superficial part of your being; your other energy bodies affect you much more strongly than your physical body.

Before embarking on sexual meditation, Taoists had potential students answer two questions. First, are you energetically willing and capable of directly communicating what's inside all your energetic bodies to your partner, capable of becoming energetically naked and intimate enough to just let the deeper parts of your being hang out there to be experienced? Second, are you willing to feel what the other person is going through on all those levels? If you are willing to fulfill these two conditions, then sexual meditation practices teach you to use sex to enter someone else's energy field and influence it. You can help them feel and release their blockages, while healing and smoothing the chi that runs between both of you, at all levels.

## SEX AT ALL STAGES OF YOUR LIFE

For most people, cultivating sexual chi is a lifetime progression because it has the potential for completely engaging and connecting the body, mind and spirit. In youth, the sexual practices help fully release the body's chi while engaging the elements of mind and spirit, which helps the process. In middle age, the emphasis becomes releasing the energy of the mind and emotions, while further engaging and connecting the body and spirit. In old age, the emphasis is on engaging the spirit, so that you become fully connected and present to yourself, which can extend to the time after you leave your physical form.

### Youth

When you are young and your sexual appetite is high, sexual chi gung fully opens up your body's chi so you can most enjoy this naturally energetic phase of human life. Sexual chi gung helps ameliorate the rage of hormones and the accompanying mood swings that can go from elation to depression. It helps remove the inner obstacles so you can get past the "I don't know what I want to do with my life syndrome." As you take advantage of the practices that open your mind, you mature faster and become less self-absorbed. Sexual chi gung can also help your first relationships to be true awakenings and experiences of growth rather than emotional rollercoaster rides. It helps you distinguish the separation between your parents and your lover. This is a big deal in the West. As you take control of your energy to help relax and survive the excesses of youth, you prepare your body and mind for the next stage of your life.

## Middle Age

Throughout history, the nature of middle age is that people enter the most productive and potentially creative times of their lives. They have gotten through the excesses of youth; they have had some education and learned to put it to use. Unfortunately, in our culture, productivity decreases for many as the amount of stress rises. The responsibilities of work, family, children and parents become overwhelming. The greatest single thing that sexual chi gung and other chi practices can do is to help you find a still place inside yourself where the responsibilities, at least internally, cease to be a burden. In the middle phase of your life, sexual meditation can be a gateway to open the heart center and to more deeply explore your relationship with your partner and the core of your being. As you become healthier in body and mind, you can protect and build the sexual energy of the body and all its mechanisms so it will last and function well into old age.

## Older Age

One of the great "secrets" of chi practices is that they help people maintain their sexual vitality well into old age. Given that half of Western society will be over fifty years of age by 2020, the myths about older people being sexually washed up and useless need a revolutionary overhaul, one that could be led by seniors. Taoist sexual practices could really come into their own because many older people might not want to give up that part of their lives just because there is another candle on their birthday cake. There is no reason why sex cannot be as rewarding and as much fun as golf and other hobbies—provided people remain mindful of sexually transmitted diseases. If older people have already learned and used chi practices to free up some of the burdens of their mental and emotional turmoil, they can choose to explore sexual meditation and fully open up their psychic, karmic and spiritual potentials. They become the wise leaders of the Chi Revolution by being comfortable with themselves and overcoming the fear of their own deaths.

## THE CHI OF SEX: RENEWABLE AND SUSTAINABLE

The good news is that cultivating your sexual energy becomes a source of renewable, sustained chi that you can cultivate well into old age. At the level of sexual chi gung, you can become healthier, more relaxed and fully open and intimate, not only with your partner but also within the depths of your own being. At the level of sexual meditation, you and your partner learn to explore your psychic, karmic and spiritual potential.

# CHAPTER 12

# Exploring Your Inner World with Prayer and Meditation

once asked Liu Hung Chieh, my main teacher and one of China's most renowned Taoist masters, why he chose not to teach Taoist meditation very often. "Not many want to learn it," was his terse response. This wise man explained that the path of spiritual evolution was far more difficult to undertake than my training in Taoist martial arts and chi gung tui na (energetic healing). Because it was a deeply important matter, Liu explained the process in detail and offered me the choice of whether or not to aspire to this journey. After serious consideration, I made the decision to follow in my teacher's path knowing full well that I would have to summon all of my courage. True to Liu's word, Taoist meditation is the most formidable yet the most fulfilling chi work I have ever encountered in my life.

## WHY MEDITATE?

If you lived in the ancient world and you walked up to most people who knew something about meditation and asked them, "Why should I meditate?" they would tell you not to meditate with that attitude. The "Why should I buy this?" attitude we often find today was not germane in those days. The idea that you're going to *get* something from meditation is actually the problem that meditation is trying to solve.

That is not to say that some very practical benefits cannot be gained from meditation. Modern science has proven that if you meditate, it will lower your blood pressure and reduce stress. It has also been shown that if you chant the mantra "Om-Coca-Cola, Om-Coca-Cola, Om-Coca-Cola," it will also lower your blood pressure. Now, I don't know what that has to do with spirituality—but if you do it, it will work.

Taoist meditation is about finding peace, joy and happiness inside yourself—that place within you where you have the energy of life and the love that actually moves through life. You will never discover freedom and stillness inside yourself from any external object, or even from the "idea" of God. Meditation is a means by which you can free yourself from the negative emotions and inner demons that tear you apart. Meditation can free you from your incessant wants and desires, which keep you spinning like a hamster in a cage. Meditation can teach you to let go of the things that you probably know you would really be better off without. Meditation allows you to integrate the experiences of your life into the core of your being, so that you are not pulled in a thousand confused directions.

Every genuine meditation tradition makes a core distinction between the external world and your inner life. Everyone has the need for an outer life—to make money, to receive an education, to find shelter. Equally important is that you need to have an inner life—some place inside where you are at peace, where your mind is stable and smooth, where your emotions are not riding you like a rollercoaster. What is it inside you that will allow you to ride out the many waves of life? How do you value, regardless of your outer life, your inner wealth? Traveling along the inner path can eventually bring you to a sense of balance, naturalness, compassion and wisdom. These are the qualities to which the Taoists aspire through meditation.

## MEDITATION, STILLNESS AND CHANGE

In many Eastern meditation methods, the goal is to achieve a deeply experienced state of inner stillness. However, in Taoist meditation, this is only a temporary, single event, immensely life-serving but not complete in and of itself.

What about the swirling infinite round of changes and difficult and unpredictable events that go on when you are not meditating and being still? No doubt, sitting on a cushion and temporarily feeling inner stillness can give you a rest and regenerative break from the unpredictable and often stressful winds of life. But if the break is only temporary, what is still can again become noisy. Spiritual practices become more complicated when you must also deal effectively with the unpredictability of what other people can do. You also have to deal with what activates inside yourself in response to that unpredictability.

A classic Eastern story describes this situation, which parallels the ancient Taoist saying: "The most enlightened Taoist sages live in town and not in the isolated countryside."

## TAOIST VIEW OF SPIRITUALITY

Most people have some belief commonly labeled as "spirituality." In Taoism, taking a spiritual path means restoring balance and becoming natural in all aspects of our lives so that we can realize our greater potential. Taoists strive for genuine compassion for themselves and others. At the most mundane level, you learn to bring balance to as much of your daily life as possible. This includes balancing the competing needs of a spiritual practice, family, personal relationships, social obligations, helping others, making money and having a satisfying life. The lack of balance in the modern, overscheduled, under-rested, thoroughly stressed world corrodes and shreds the joy of living.

At a spiritual level, balance means first acquiring a baseline of

## The Holy Man Goes to Town

After many, many years of practice, a holy man meditates alone on top of a mountain. He appears enlightened, as nothing disturbs his peace of mind.

Then he decides to leave the mountain and live in town. He reckons if his spirit is truly stable and clear, he can smoothly engage with the hustle and bustle of urban daily life. After a short time, the holy man becomes agitated and eventually blows up from having to deal with all the disturbing people, unpredictable variables and chaotic situations.

Being a genuine spiritual seeker who also wants to succeed in daily life, he recognizes that his self-perceived spiritual stability was false—a pleasant self-delusion but an illusion nevertheless. So he goes back to the mountain to overcome the blockages that disturbed him. When he regains peace of mind, he goes back to town. Alas, other problems emerge and again, he has to go back to his mountain to overcome them. He practices until his spirit remains clear and open in his daily life in town, with all the ups and downs of life's infinite variety of internal experiences.

internal stillness inside. Gradually you obtain and integrate the different levels of peak experiences or super-conscious states, called "emptiness." At its highest level, this is also known as the "great stillness." As you experience progressively stronger states of awareness and emptiness, you go deeper and deeper toward your essence, the seventh energy body. There you will find the natural flow of your core, your essence beyond the stories of your history or personality. Eventually you arrive at true balance, which leads to complete spiritual clarity, wisdom, and smoothness with both the seen and unseen world. Within the waters of achieving deep inner balance and stillness, the seeds of compassion grow and flourish from the depths of your being.

For Taoists, compassion implies a willingness to impartially love and extend positive energy to everything and everyone. Compassion implies a willingness to forgive everything in life—starting with yourself—for anything and everything that has happened or might happen. The proverb, "Everything furthers," urging compassion, echoes like a constant, drum-like refrain in the *I Ching*.

Spiritual beings—at the innermost center of their souls—recognize the common threads that unite rather than separate the "me, us and them" boundaries of tribal identities. You must make a conscious effort to shift your innermost identity from one that centers primarily on the good or self-interests of you or your tribe. The focus is on the good of the whole, in harmony with universal love and compassion. You aspire to treat everyone as well as you can, whether you know someone or the person is a stranger. You do not selectively treat some people well just because they are members of your tribe, family, religion, color or any other discrimination for which you could conceive. Nor do you justify treating others poorly because they are not members of your tribe. The more spiritually asleep people are, the more they live within narrow tribal boundaries unable to recognize the energy of life.

## LIVING MEDITATION

The word "meditation" in our modern, educated culture has come to mean virtually nothing. People say they meditate and, if they just say that, it sounds wonderful. But you don't actually know what it is they do.

Jesus Christ said the kingdom of heaven is in your own heart. The doorway to that kingdom is genuine prayer or meditation. All the great religious leaders meditated. Many of their followers did as well, their prayers coming from deep within themselves. Today, however, people talk about a belief in God rather than their experience of God; instead of prayers that come from within, they have recitations or intellectual, internal dialogues with themselves. Meditation and prayer help you connect with the deep kingdom of spirituality within yourself—*ruah,* the ancient Hebrew and Aramaic word for spirit.

Some people meditate on prosperity, on visualizing wealth, but this has little to do with an inner life. Others confuse meditation with contemplation. They think about an idea and that becomes meditating on an idea. From an Eastern point of view, that's not meditation; it's analysis. Still others think about how it is they should be thinking, how they should be living their lives, which is more a study in philosophy. Taoist meditation is not *thinking* about something. It is being able to release the chi that is attached to any thought or any emotion—the ability to let go.

Self-love, loving oneself, is one of the common topics of discussion in the West. Why? Because many people believe that there is something fundamentally wrong with themselves and they feel little self-worth. At a very deep level, they do not like themselves. The Taoists used meditation to deal with removing everything that keeps you from loving yourself. I've developed a system for teaching these Taoist techniques, which I call TAO meditation. It changes the deepest substructures of your mind, your soul or your spirit, so you will discover stability at the core of your being. There, you become at peace and in balance from within. If you take away all that is false, all you will be left with is that which is true: naturalness, deep awareness and compassion. You are not trying to understand yourself; that's a thought process. TAO meditation will actually enable you to completely release the chi of your thoughts, body, emotions and karma. This is the realistic process of cultivating love and compassion in all the moments of your life.

## THE DISSOLVING METHOD

As with all chi practices the process of TAO meditation entails two basic steps. The first asks you to go inside your body, mind and spirit and recognize where chi blockages reside at progressively deeper levels. The second part asks you to release the chi blockages, a process known as the Inner Dissolving method, passed down by Lao Tse over 2,500 years ago. The Chi Scanning exercise in the Chi Rev Workout will help you build the foundation for later practicing the Inner Dissolving method of meditation.[1] This progression occurs in your first seven energy bodies, clearing blockages one by one into emptiness. As you free each layer, the process gets deeper and more challenging at the physical, energetic, emotional and mental levels because you are working with the subtler, less obvious energies that we don't normally experience in daily life. At the level of the psychic, karmic and spiritual energy bodies, you are working more intensely with the subtle energies of the unseen world.

All chi exercises will activate chi blockages in ways that physical, cardiovascular exercise cannot. Stored and bound energy and the attached potential—subliminal memories—can be triggered during energetic exercises. Rather than remaining suppressed and relatively quiet, these energies bubble up into your conscious awareness and become very loud. At this point you have effectively afforded yourself the opportunity to resolve, rather than ignore, that which binds and compresses you, once and for all.

---

[1] The author's complete meditation course, *The TAO of Letting Go* (six-CD set), will help you take the next step and actually begin the Inner Dissolving method.

*A little over seven months ago I was diagnosed with liver cancer. I was greatly afraid of the threat of death looming over me.*

*Since then, Bruce's CD,* The TAO of Letting Go, *teaching the basic principles of TAO meditation, has been my faithful companion. Initially, I used the practices to help me get over the shock of the diagnosis. Since then, they have helped me face the most important challenges of my life.*

*I listened to the section on fear. As I tuned into the layers of my fears, I was able to gradually let go. I learned how to deal with the possibility of my nonexistence in a relaxed way, which in turn has freed me up to live life more fully, stay focused on what I needed to do to heal and be on my way to a cure.*

*A few months later, I had an operation called a chemo-embolization without any anesthesia or meds. Before the operation I listened to the CD for three and a half hours, using it to go into a deeper and deeper meditation. When the doctors operated, if there was the least amount of pain, I used the Dissolving method to go even deeper. I could differentiate actual sensations from the negative charges of the past and my fear of the future. As I did so, I also released some past traumas and shocks, a nice perk. I have found a way to comfortably relinquish some of my many beloved activities and habits, and my ego, and let go of many of the things that I did not need.*

*Six months later, I attended Bruce's summer workshop. Although I was not wholly cured, I felt healed and fully alive. The most important thing I have learned is how to integrate all the issues and events I experience every day so I feel connected to myself and the universe, which enables me to become calmer, more focused and productive. Today, I have a much higher probability of living longer, while growing, thriving and enjoying my life more fully.*

—Richard Amarnick
Newton, Massachusetts

# QUALITIES OF CHI BLOCKAGES

The process of identifying chi blockages requires you to find enough stability and stillness inside yourself to focus inside your body. The Chi Rev Workout has introduced you to some of the chi exercises that can lead you to a still point. Fundamental to TAO meditation is the ability to recognize and resolve these blockages. TAO meditation teaches you to begin noticing where chi is agitated or disturbed and to become present to the experience of that blockage. Once you discover a blockage, you release it until you arrive at the point of emptiness and inner stillness, where all blockages become resolved and healed.

All chi blockages have one or more of four distinct qualities that were introduced in Chapter 5: tension; strength; something that doesn't feel quite right, especially if you don't know what it is; and any kind of contraction. Most chi practices teach you to begin by putting your attention on the top of your head, regardless of whether you are standing, sitting, moving or lying down, or whether or not you are in relationship to someone else, as is the case with sparring, verbal conversation or sex. Next, with your mind and intent, you focus inward and scan slowly downward, looking for any of the four qualities that will identify a chi blockage.

## Tension

Tension always involves a struggle; something is seeking dominance over something else. Tension could reside in the muscles as they pull against each other. Your thoughts could cause tension, such as the complexity of a task and the amount of time you have to complete it. You could have emotional tension, such as anger or fear, which draws your attention from positive emotions and observations.

## Strength

Strength has a whole different meaning in meditation than feeling powerful, whether in the muscles or in the mind. In TAO meditation, it means the strength attached to the ego, the controlling one that says, "This is what I will do; I will make the world be the way I want it to be; I will deal with my problems no matter how difficult by blasting and pushing through them." Strength is about being unable to let go of fixations and beliefs, a way of producing a restriction inside you. When your energy is balanced and flowing smoothly, you don't feel strong. You feel comfortable, loose and natural without the necessity for force. You can go with the flow.

## Something that Does Not Feel Quite Right— Especially if You Don't Know What It Is

These are the deepest memories you have from life-altering experiences. They might even include your time in the womb or even the first six months of childhood when you were incapable of registering language. People are recorders, picking up and storing every input they receive throughout life. You might not be able to recall every circumstance, but all past events have been integrated and have helped shape you into the person you are today. We register such inputs as negative energy coming from a parent or accumulated karma deep in our DNA. We lock them somewhere in the nervous system or brain without being conscious of it or even assenting to it. Something that doesn't feel quite right typically lies below your conscious radar and gives you an uneasy feeling for which you can't necessarily identify a cause. Just because there is no telling exactly where this feeling comes from does not mean it is false. So learning to recognize the quality of something that does not feel quite right and allowing ourselves to be present to the experience itself is important in TAO meditation.

## Contraction

The presence or absence of this quality differentiates someone who is very awake and open from someone who is sleepwalking through life and has closed down. When people are stressed or fearful, the body shuts down and contracts—blood vessels constrict, internal organs downgrade their performance, the breath is held. So rather than the chi of any of your first seven energy bodies being open and flowing, it is contracted and shut down. A thousand diseases of the body/mind can be attributed to little more than something in the body closing down. This is the definition of a heart attack, isn't it? A big artery closes down. Depression? The brain shows decreased neural activity. Kidney or liver failure? The organs don't work as efficiently to keep pace with the larger system. Chronic fatigue syndrome? The body doesn't have the energy to sustain itself through the day. Carpal tunnel syndrome? The joints become stiff and lack flexibility and range of motion. Taoists attribute contraction to the power of the ego and believe it to be the hallmark of death.

## RELEASING BLOCKAGES

Once you can recognize where chi is blocked, you must learn how to release it so that it does not keep coming back at you like a boomerang. Hate and resentment are like a curved blade that, when harbored, come back to cut their bearer. TAO meditation is renowned for the methods that teach you to release that which blocks and binds you so you can be free from the inside. Taoists call this process the Dissolving method, for which Chi Scanning—the second exercise in the Chi Rev Workout discussed in detail in Chapter 17—is the preparatory or outer phase. The metaphor used for millennia is "ice to water; water to gas" (Outer Dissolving), or "ice to water; water to space" (Inner Dissolving). Ice is the blockage, frozen inside you; as the blockage begins to dissolve, it turns metaphorically into a liquid as it softens and relaxes, finally in Outer Dissolving turning into a gas that disperses into thin air. This completes the release at the boundary of your aura beyond your skin. In Inner Dissolving you release into inner space deep inside your body, where the depths of your being or soul lives. At that point, the blockage fully dissolves and simply vanishes from your body, mind and spirit. Chi is then free to flow smoothly and powerfully as it did when you were an infant.

## ENERGETIC TRAINING IN TAO MEDITATION

Intellectually, the process of recognizing and dissolving chi blockages might sound straightforward and relatively easy. You will not become enlightened overnight, however. If the process were so easy, a lot more enlightened beings would be roaming the planet!

First, just as I did, you have to decide whether you really want to confront and free yourself of everything that binds you or remain in some state of denial. The choice is yours: Consider taking some time to answer this question carefully, because there is no point in trying to excel at a skill that you honestly do not care to practice.

Second, you have to be willing to commit time, every day, to your

## Ice to Water; Water to Gas

To get a sense of the power of the Dissolving method, clench your fist as tightly as you can. Your energy begins to contract within a few seconds and the blood will flow out of your hand until your knuckles turn white. The energy is now frozen like ice. When you open your fist, the energy comes back into the hand along with the blood—ice to water. Next, focus your awareness on your hand until it completely relaxes and feels almost empty of all solidity, like air, and becomes quite comfortable—water to gas.

This process can go on for several years as you work through recognizing and dissolving all the blockages in your seven energy bodies. Notice how you can become more aware of the subtleties of both the tightening and the releasing phase of the experiment.

chi practice and develop a regular rhythm. Chi exercises, when done as daily practices, have been proven to be effective for thousands of years. However, you cannot aspire to deal with the large issues that directly affect the state of your health, emotions, mind and karma if you are not fully committed to your practice.

Third, you will want to use exercises such as tai chi and chi gung to develop the courage and stability to face the deeper and multi-faceted demons you might confront in your meditation practice. These exercises can help you build a strong foundation.

Finally, you must be willing to relax, let go and give up control. Chi exercises, such as TAO yoga, will help you if you can make them a rhythm of your daily life. Taoists are fond of the phrase "separate and combine." Learn and stabilize one aspect of your practice first before folding it into or combining it seamlessly with a more sophisticated practice method.

## THE FIVEFOLD PATH: BODY-ENERGY-SPIRIT-EMPTINESS-TAO

The three treasures of Taoism, *jing-chi-shen* in Chinese and *body-energy-spirit* in English, must be developed in order to aspire to emptiness, and finally realization of the TAO. Emptiness is the birthing ground of change. For true emptiness to emerge, the flow between ever-changing conditions and emptiness is essential. Emptiness allows true stability and naturalness of the mind and essence of the human spirit to emerge. The ability to fluidly move in harmony with all the ways in which change can occur is embodied in the *I Ching*—the book of changes—which lies at the heart of Taoism.

As you do your chi practices, you will find that much of what you learn will seep into the activities of your daily life. Eventually, you could aspire to bringing your consciousness to every moment and become truly present to your experiences. Truly moving toward life is the energy behind the Chi Revolution.

# CHAPTER 13

# The *I Ching*: The Mother Lode of the Chi Revolution

The *I Ching* is commonly referred to as some sort of super oracle. Some "throw" the *I Ching* to help make decisions or to gain insight into the future. That's what twentieth-century visionary psychiatrist Carl Jung saw the *I Ching* to be when he was asked to write the foreword to one of the most popular translations.[1] It is what a lot of hippies did in the sixties and seventies. Like astrology, it gave them a new vocabulary and context with which to examine themselves, their relationships and their dreams.

The reason it worked so well as a divination tool, at least from a Western perspective, is that the book's language is fairly nebulous and allegorical, although from a Taoist perspective it is not. The first thing that happens when you throw the *I Ching* is that you ask a question, and the message that comes up is meant to open your conscious mind. However, the clarity of the message you get depends very much on first taking the time to make yourself quiet and internally stable. If you are noisy or distracted, you will not get a clear message. In this way, the second thing that happens when

---

[1] *I Ching or Book of Changes: The Richard Wilhelm Translation* rendered into English by Cary F. Baynes (Bollingen Foundation, 1950).

you throw the *I Ching* is that it becomes a psychic conduit between you and an energetic source or the chi of the universe. It gives you an access channel to your personal, human intuition.

## TAOISM AND THE *I CHING*

Few people realize that the *I Ching* lies at the root of Taoism and could be considered its bible. This is not surprising since many things that are basic to Chinese culture aren't known very well in the West, although some pragmatic applications, such as acupuncture and tai chi, are beginning to filter into modern culture. China's difficult and impenetrable society, the language barrier and distrust of foreigners are the main reasons why many Westerners still harbor misconceptions or lack knowledge of China's sophisticated traditions even after all this time. The fundamental principles of Taoism originated from an intimate and thorough understanding of the *I Ching*. My teacher taught me the *I Ching* in three steps—this is what it says; this is what it means; and this is how to do it—first through chi practices and later through integrating the principles into my daily activities. The Taoists recognized that inherent to change is its power to destroy anyone who does not possess balance, compassion and naturalness. Balance is essential for compassion and naturalness to arise, so you start by attempting to balance all eight energy bodies. You start physically with chi exercises, such as tai chi, chi gung and TAO yoga, to clear blockages and make the body stable. As we've discussed, this process goes through all the energy bodies, each layer getting progressively deeper and more expansive.

## THE MOTHER LODE OF YIN AND YANG

There are two levels of intent in everything you do in chi practices. The first one is ordinary intent. Any intent has both a yin and yang component. If you want to walk across the street, that's a yang action because you have to go and do something. If you want something to come toward you, that's a yin form of intent. But then there are these questions: Where does the intent come from to begin with? Where do all your thoughts come from? Where do all your emotions come from? Where is the birthing room of yin and yang? This is the second level of intent, the place from which intent arises originally—where intent is born.

Classic Chinese philosophy says that in the beginning there was the undifferentiated void called *wu chi (wu ji)*. Wu chi held within itself all possibilities but was beyond needing to take form. However, in order for creation to come into existence, a creative force was needed. This force was called *tai chi (taiji)*. The words "tai" and "chi" encompass two philosophical and spiritual concepts. Tai means large or great; chi or ji (in this context, pronounced like the "gee" of "gee whiz") connotes the superlative of a word, such as biggest, richest, deepest. It is not the same as the word chi used in this book, which means life-force energy. So here, tai chi or taiji is usually translated as "the great supreme."

Tai chi gives birth to yin and yang. Tai chi is neutral, including either one, neither and both. Although it has no specific qualities of its own, it allows any yin and yang to take form. It is a level of emptiness that produces manifestation.

Out of the empty tai chi comes the interplay of yin and yang, which is called *liang i (liang yi)* by the ancient Chinese. So, where does any thought, any emotion, any phenomena come from? If you have a psychic perception, where does it come from? If a thought comes into your mind, or an emotion comes into your body, where does it originate? The thought itself, the emotion itself, the psychic perception itself or even the way karma occurs itself you could say always has a yin or a yang quality. It could be more yin and less yang or more yang and less yin, but one or both are always involved. You can break anything down from the smallest particles that exist in quantum physics to the biggest things in the universe. All have a yin and yang component.

## A Map of the Energetic Universe

For Taoists, the *I Ching* is a map that represents how the energy of the universe works. It is about how opposites in the universe—yin and yang—combine, interact and differentiate to represent energy in both the seen and the unseen worlds. In the *I Ching*, chi is represented by sixty-four hexagrams that contain combinations of unbroken yang lines and broken yin lines, which create all the possibilities of how opposites can interact with each other. So you could say that the *I Ching* represents the possibilities of life in the universe, anytime, anyplace, anywhere. The *I Ching*'s cosmology is remarkably similar to the way the sixty-four strands of DNA, the molecule of life, pair and entwine to form double helixes. Similarly, zeros and ones pair to form the basis of computer codes for software programs. All are source codes to the trillions of combinations that can result.

There are lots of theories out there about who authored the *I Ching*, but no one really knows where it came from. We do know that it has no single, definable author and that its principles existed

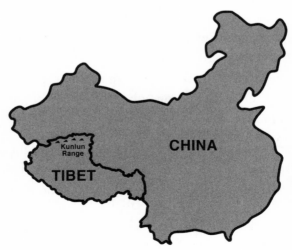

*Map of Tibet and the Kunlun Mountains*

as an oral tradition for over 8,000 years. Oral tradition speculates that the text might have migrated over to China from the Kunlun Mountains between northern Tibet and the Takla Makan Desert (see map on p. 120).

## CONTINUITY OF CHANGE

If there is anything true in our lives, in history, in the life of the universe and solar system, it is that everything is always in flux. Chi is always in flux, constantly changing. So another way Taoists consider the *I Ching* is as an allegorical language or code about how change works in the universe. In the *I Ching*, change is represented by the way energy continually changes from a straight line, which is a beginning or yang force, and a broken line, which is an end or yin force. This concept applies to the way changing chi is embedded in most metaphysical subjects to the ways in which chi permeates all the techniques of any chi practice, including the ones you do alone, such as tai chi or chi gung, and those that others do to you, such as acupuncture or chi gung tui na. All these applications come from the *I Ching*.

On the deepest levels, as you become incredibly relaxed and at ease with yourself, chi practices can help you to accept changes in your life and to become able to flow smoothly with them. And, as with all chi practices, study of the *I Ching* over a long period will create a much deeper understanding of the forces of chi in yourself and in the universe.

Most people, however, do not undertake this study. My teacher Liu Hung Chieh put it really well when he said most people just want to learn how to flip the switch to turn on a light bulb. Only a very small percentage of people will actually want to understand how the electrical system is wired or how to build power plants and create electrical grids. Most people just want to learn simple chi practices that could make a difference in their lives. They don't necessarily want to know exactly how chi flows inside them or in the universe. Very few people become interested in how chi really works, where they can take it in their lives or how far it can take them.

## The Flow Between Movement and Stillness

It is not enough to recognize that all the thinking processes and events of life are impermanent and subject to never-ending changes. There need to be practical methods to embody this concept within yourself and to make it real for you. Otherwise the classic bedrock phrase of Taoism and Buddhism, "Stillness is movement and movement is stillness" seems mere hollow talk, which it most certainly is not. The flow between movement and stillness permeates every chi practice and is the heart of the *I Ching*.

The empty space in the middle of the trigrams of the *I Ching* represents the great emptiness, the universal chi that gives birth to all and everything from thought to the infinite galaxies, stars and planets in the majesty of the night sky. Around this empty space, the eight trigrams represent the matrix behind all the changes that can manifest in the universe from the gross to the most subtle.

Long before the historical Buddha Shakyamuni was born, Taoists arrived at the meaning of what has been adopted as a phrase of both Buddhism and Taoism, "Emptiness is Form and Form is Emptiness."

For true emptiness to emerge into human awareness, the flow between change or movement—represented by the changing nature of the trigrams—and emptiness (or stillness)—represented by the empty space—must intertwine. For true stability and naturalness of mind and essence to emerge, there must be a seamless, unimpeded flow of energy and spirit. This aspect, which lies at the heart of Taoism and all its practices is embodied throughout the *I Ching*.

## Why Throw the *I Ching*?

The purpose of the *I Ching* is to give you insights into life's dance with chi. Throwing the *I Ching* might help you understand:

- The yin-yang nature of change so you can flow through it rather than crashing into it with great stress and dissonance.
- Wu chi and tai chi—the space in the middle from which all things are derived; the Buddhists would say this is the relationship between the relative (yin and yang) and the absolute (wu chi/tai chi).
- What is changeable and what is not; there are hundreds of chi practices for helping you understand this—the classical one being ba gua—an internal martial art.

At any moment, the substratum, from which everything emerges, has a flow pattern. The *I Ching* allows you to tap into this substratum and activate it inside you so you can have some internal clarity about your life and move with it instead of going in the opposite direction.

## How to Throw the *I Ching*

It is ideal to have someone else throw the *I Ching* for you so that your question can be answered objectively. In fact, if someone who knows you well throws the stalks or coins on your behalf, he or she could be just as subjective as you. So, at the very least, you should not share the question with the person who throws the coins or stalks. Others do not have to be knowledgeable about the *I Ching* to do this for you.

Prepare yourself by arriving at a calm, still state. If you can, your conscious awareness should enter your central channel—the place where all your thoughts can go to quiet and peace.[1] Next, let your intuition flow toward the unseen world with surrender. Go quiet for at least a minute although some do this for up to an hour. Now you're prepared to throw the *I Ching*. You are looking for something from the substratum that is not knowable; you do not throw the *I Ching* for something you can figure out yourself. You throw it when have no way of knowing what is going to emerge and morph downstream.

Go into the substratum and stay there until you feel everything opening up. You have no agenda, yet you feel a sense of the flux.

---

[1] The central channel is discussed in the author's book, *Opening the Energy Gates of Your Body*.

At that stage of the game, you throw the yarrow stalks or coins. The stalks are preferred since there could be some subconscious skill in throwing two-sided coins. Any good edition of the *I Ching* will explain exactly how to throw the sticks, create your hexagram and locate the corresponding descriptions that explain the meaning of your formation in regard to the question you posed. In this way, the manner in which you construct your question is crucially important to the answer you will receive.

The trigrams found in the *I Ching* represent complex, dynamic combinations of continuous yin and yang changes. One of the oldest chi practices is walking the ba gua circle, a method of moving meditation that existed side by side with the sitting Taoist meditation practices.[1] In the *I Ching*, the primary or essential energies of the universe are represented by the ba gua or eight trigrams (*ba*—eight; *gua*—trigram). Once the sticks are thrown and you figure out the patterns of the lines, there is a brief moment, a gasp or an "aack," that follows. Just let your mind go very quiet and sink into the substratum. Sync with the substratum.

Finally, you read the appropriate descriptions in the *I Ching*. What is supposed to come up, or what can come up, will. Let your awareness go to trying to get to the place from which the changes are coming. The *I Ching* is one such focal point.

## WALKING THE CIRCLE TO UNDERSTAND CHANGE

There is change—incessant change. In the current era, the world is evolving at a rate previously unknown in human history. Reliance on computers, advances in science and population growth contribute to the inability of people to prepare for change. Human beings are forced to adapt tens of thousands of years ahead of their evolutionary capacity. Anxiety is the disease of the modern age because we cannot keep up. Human beings become rigid and fearful when forced to give up their securities.

---

[1] The circle walking method is taught in detail in the author's TAO meditation book, *The Great Stillness*.

Chi practices, such as the ancient practice of walking the ba gua circle, help people cope with and accept change. There is a whole art to practicing until you simply relax, accept that change exists and go with the flow. Since there is no bigger change than going from moving fluidly—either slowly or at lightning speed—to being still, you first practice this on the physical level. It is said that circle walking was developed by monks some 4,000 years ago in the Kunlun Mountains north of Tibet for three intertwined purposes. The first was to achieve stillness of mind. The second was to generate a healthy, disease-free body with relaxed nerves and great stamina, which the monks needed for daily work and prolonged meditation. The third was to develop and maintain balance internally while either their inner world or the events of the external world changed.

Over time, the physical practices of ba gua, as well as chi gung, become a metaphor for your meditation practice. You learn to apply the same skill, precision and techniques to addressing your emotional, psychic and karmic bodies as you have in your physical practice. If you internally fixate or internally disconnect, you cannot go with the flow. Eventually, when you lose your resistance to change, you can. This is a primary goal of all chi practices, such as ba gua, chi gung and even tai chi, although in different ways. You can explore the chi flow at all levels of the energy bodies and all sublayers therein. As a ba gua practitioner becomes more and more developed internally and externally, he or she can experience spontaneous movement during circle walking, which frees deeply bound spiritual energies.

## WHOLENESS AND SPIRITUALITY

The *I Ching* is a channel for becoming whole inside ourselves rather than being disconnected or split into many fragments. At the end of the day, when the energies inside a human being are harmonious and balanced with each other, they will make that person feel whole. If they are out of balance, a human being will feel incredibly stressed at the level of their body, mind and emotions, which can result in a myriad of diseases. Further, at a very fundamental spiritual level, the light inside them just does not shine. Instead of feeling smooth from the stability generated by their inner world, they feel shaky, confused and fractionated. They become prone to fixating on external factors.

On the deeper level of spirituality, the energies that connect with our inner world are the same energies used for contacting and communicating with other souls beyond the boundaries of time and space. Taoists were interested in the ways in which beings can contact the essences of other people. The study of the *I Ching* takes you back to the source of spirituality that pervades all and everything. That is why the center of the *I Ching* symbol is empty. There's nothing there. And that emptiness, the undifferentiated void, *wu chi,* was considered by the Taoists to be that which held the force, *tai chi,* of all the possibilities of manifestation in existence, beyond needing to take any form itself.

## STILLNESS ALONE MAY NOT BE ENOUGH

The *I Ching* provides the roots of the Chi Revolution: *jing-chi-shen-wu-TAO.* The ability to cope with change is what all chi practices help you develop. The benefits to our lives are immeasurable. How much is your health worth to you? And, if you are healthy or develop the ability to self-heal, is there a larger purpose? If you consider the Taoist perspective, anything less than complete spiritual awakening is a lack of complete spiritual health. For Taoists, being enlightened is to be spiritually healthy.

The study of the *I Ching* provides the foundation for strengthening the spiritual potential inside yourself. It is the opening of your capacity to move toward the potential realization of life—toward emptiness. However, all chi practices give you the ability to feel and strengthen your chi as well as discover how yin and yang interact within you, with others, with the space we share, the planet we inhabit and the whole universe. This includes the chi that makes our bodies function; the way our emotions interact, change and move around each other; the weaving of our thoughts and their connections with others; and the way we can perceive and even be active in the psychic world, the unseen world and the karmic world.

## RIDING THE WAVES OF CHANGE

On a practical level, the Chi Revolution is about how chi practices have the power to impact our existence as human beings. It is about the ways chi moves inside and affects us; the effects of our thoughts and emotions; the expansive, creative and positive forces in ourselves and others; and about the energy around us becoming genuinely smooth and nourishing for a deep, inherent sense of life around us. Sometimes I take my students to the ocean, lead them into a still state and ask them to see if they can feel one or more of the eight energy bodies. First I talk about how the waves they see are generated by forces deep within the ocean. For Taoists, waves are a classical representation of change. If we can tap into the large reservoirs beneath those waves, which are the same within us, we can learn that change is just the ebb and flow of energy.

The *I Ching* is about exploring possibilities, discovering what is, being comfortable with it and then having the capacity to move with the ebb and flow of the tides.

CHAPTER 14

# The Law of Return: Accessing Your Karma with Chi

Have you ever felt drawn toward someone without a conscious thought as to why? Have you ever met someone for the first time and immediately sensed a strong connection? Perhaps you harbored ill will toward someone for no particular reason that went beyond any identifiable stereotypes. On the surface, these encounters might appear to be random. Yet there is something in these interactions that point to an inherent destiny. Your personal experience might have a larger context. One possibility is that what you are experiencing could be of a karmic nature. Although knowledge about karma has been held for thousands of years, the teachings have rarely been shared with Westerners. Traditionally the knowledge was held in closed monasteries or temples in the East, reserved only for those people who were interested in completing their final incarnation, something that Western living tends to interrupt.

## LINKING CHI TO KARMA

The word karma is often thrown around quite unconsciously. People say, "We must have had a past life together," or "I must have been royalty in a past life." Maybe this is true and maybe it's not. Most of the time, these statements are mental thoughts, abstract ideas that are not necessarily based upon reality and have no bearing on your current life in any case. However, they do speak to the underlying consciousness of the energy behind life. The great secret is this: Chi is the link between you and your karma.

As discussed in Chapter 3, the sixth energy body is called the causal or karmic body. As you develop the ability to feel and work with chi, eventually you can reach a point where you access karma.

Why would someone want to consider their karma? At the base level, it is important for people to become aware of the effect they have on others and the effects others have on them. The spirit of "what goes around comes around" is universally recognized, but there are much deeper and more significant forces at play. At the more advanced levels, a person can consciously and directly consider karmic debts one by one, and possibly resolve them. In fact, karma is one of the reasons we are on this planet in a human body.

## THE NATURE OF KARMA

From the point of view of Buddhists and Hindus, karma, a Sanskrit word, is defined as cause and effect. Once energy goes out in any direction, it always returns to itself. In this view, if energy goes out as good, it would return as good. If energy goes out as evil, it returns as evil. If energy goes out as confusion, it comes back to create more confusion. These effects could occur immediately or over a long period, such as over many lifetimes. If you want to test the cause-effect relationship of karma, do this: For two days, smile and only say kind things to everyone you greet. Carefully observe the ways in which people treat you. Then do the opposite for two days—insult every person you greet. And watch how they react.

You could say that you attract certain energies to yourself because of the karma you put out. If you punch someone in the face, that person will most likely punch you back—maybe literally, maybe figuratively. You can say this is karma, but in the Taoist view, it is not the whole story.

## THE TAOIST LAW OF RETURN

Taoists do not actually use the term karma. They talk about the Law of Return. For Taoists, all energy flows in a circle. On this, contemporary physicists and Taoists agree. Energy can neither be created nor destroyed. It just keeps changing forms as it travels through specific cycles in circular energetic patterns based on the intent that is manifested. Recall that any level of intent has both a yin and yang component. In a yin cycle, energy is moving toward or being absorbed by something. In a yang cycle, energy is emanating or moving away from something. According to the Taoists, karmic energy goes out from some origination point and returns to itself in some fashion. By the time the energy returns, it has become changed and might not resemble the quality of the energy that went out. Very often, the exact qualities of its journey cannot be ascertained. The Taoists say that one of the possibilities—but only one—is that the karmic energy might come back in the way it originated. Bouncing a ball against a wall and having it bounce straight back to you is an example. But that is only one possibility. A strong gust of wind may come and blow that ball in either direction or it might be blown away altogether. More likely, in the Taoist perspective, karmic energy is moving throughout the universe. You become a particular focal point where karma moves through you and thereby causes an effect in you or others around you, an effect that might or might not be connected to your own current, obvious, recognizable actions.

Often when people talk about karma, they assign positive or negative interpretations of events as resulting from a perceived good or bad action, respectively. However, the karmic energy that attached itself to you and becomes bound inside you might have nothing to do with the energy you put out. It might have more to do with much larger flows in the universe that just happen to cross your path. These flows could have started while you and I were not even guests on this planet. So, you could say that the Law of Return has three properties:

○ All energy runs in a circle.
○ Any energetic movement has a yin and yang component, or intent, which determines whether energy is expanding outward or being absorbed inward.
○ The energy going out always returns to the origination point, but not necessarily in the same form or time frame in which it went out.

## TYPES OF KARMIC INFLUENCES

Think of karma as a carrier wave. To have an effect, it must intersect with another carrier wave to manifest some sort of consequence, whether inside you or in the universe. For example, the basis of astrology is that a carrier wave in the stars intersects with some-thing inside you and creates an effect within your personality or character that strongly influences how you will react to some external event or internal thought process. It is the intersection that causes a manifestation. In the karmic view, the context of your life and your external circumstances determines, to a certain degree, how a karmic wave is going to move inside you and consequently affect you.

So, the good news is that not everything you interpret as being of negative consequence is actually a direct result of your own "bad" actions or character. What happens could just as likely be a result of the karma of the family or nation you were born into or even the karma of the entire human race. It may have nothing to do with you personally—you may simply be an impartial catalyst for larger events downstream. Conversely, when good things happen, it may or may not have to do with your personal qualities of goodness in your character. There might be some element of luck involved.

The temptation is to use the term "random energy," but it is not random in the grand scheme of things, even though it might often seem to be the case for you personally. Almost everyone is caught up in larger waves of karmic cycles.

## FORGET WHY FOR PEACE OF MIND

The agent through which karma manifests inside you is chi. Karma is bound or blocked chi. If chi were not bound, there would be no karma. The Taoists say that trying to unravel why chi is blocked in any energy body or why something did or did not happen is a waste of time. For that, you need a fortune teller. Simply knowing the why of an event isn't going to resolve or free the blockage that is trapped inside you. What is important is to first recognize and deal directly with the karmic energy of the blockage, to dissolve that energy completely so that it cannot continue to attract other karmic energies.

If you are on a torture table, do you want to figure out how and why you got there, or do you simply want to get off the table? Attaching too deeply to the cause is to feed the blockage, not get rid of it. The thoughts will continue to torture you. To free yourself of your karmic blockages, you need to go to the core of who you are as a human being, whatever the circumstances might be in your life. If you can find out who you are without the external circumstances, you might be able to reach your essence. However, you cannot really get there until you first release and resolve the chi blockages in your karma.

## BECOMING A MATURE HUMAN BEING

Freeing your karma is the nature of TAO meditation, which is a spiritual journey. To begin this journey, you must first become a mature human being. You must become physically, emotionally and mentally stable and balanced within yourself so that you have

enough inner strength to deal with your karma. You need to develop
the ability to build up, store and harness the healing power of your
chi and employ the methods that will clear out the blockages
attached in your physical, emotional, mental and psychic bodies.

The purpose of tai chi, chi gung and other chi-movement practices
is to establish stabilized, coherent and balanced chi inside you so that
you can embark on the more difficult spiritual path of freeing yourself from your karma in meditation. Your body, mind and emotions
must be strong for you to have the courage and stamina to conquer
the more hidden, and potentially darker, karmic blockages. You need
to become internally balanced so the negative pressures of ordinary
life can no longer destabilize or crush you when confronting your
ever-darker sides.

Becoming a mature human being naturally comes before going
on to becoming a spiritual, enlightened one. From balance, the
ability to actualize love and compassion naturally flows. You must
have compassion for yourself before you can fully have compassion
for others. As compassion naturally begins to flow, you begin to
recognize the infinite connections of all life. Even if you have the
most direct, piercing insight into the core of any given situation and
the relationship to your essence, you have to clear enough of the
blockages in your physical, emotional, mental and psychic energy
bodies so you do not become frozen—so you can use that insight to
clear the blockages. Likewise, if your karma is incredibly blocked
or not fully resolved, you are less likely to reach the point of having
that insight in the first place.

## SEEING THE WHOLE

Unraveling and balancing the karmic energy that lies within many
individuals is at the core of the Chi Revolution. It is one of the final
paths to becoming liberated and enlightened in Taoism, Hinduism
and Buddhism. Resolving your karma allows you to have spiritual
peace inside yourself and flow smoothly with the universe. When a

lot of your individual karma is resolved, you see unambiguously and move effortlessly toward solutions that really work. One of the fundamental insights arising from this clarity is that you move toward a way of life that is good both for the whole and its part— for yourself. Once you have healed yourself, you can turn some of your efforts outside yourself toward healing the world. Regardless of the religious principles to which you aspire, the energy of your karma has to be addressed before you can address healing the world.

For example, the definition of a good leader is someone who actively clears his or her inner world through a regular meditative and energetic practice. In the East, they call such a person a "Sage King" (or "Sage Queen"). At the most elemental level of their life energy, these people are moving away from corruption. They are moving toward coherence rather than incoherence. They are moving toward sanity rather than insanity. It is not about their specific religious principles; it is about their concern for where life is going, what adds value to the life force and what is good for the whole.

Remember, there are two primary directions both in one's own life and the world in general—toward more life or more death— that are moved by intent and actions. The flow is never static; it always tends to move significantly in one direction or the other. A good leader would more consistently choose the direction of life over that of death.

## KARMIC RUTS IN THE UNIVERSE

Getting rid of karmic chi blockages in the universe is a much larger issue. From the perspective of a planetary scale, there's an immense amount of unresolved karma among us. When you consider all the useless wars that have been fought throughout history, it's clear that humankind still has not figured out alternative tactics even with dramatic advances in science and technology. Getting sucked into the energy of military solutions is characteristic of the ruts that people from all civilizations continue generating. It's one example of a significant karmic rut.

When karma is blocked in large groups of individuals, a larger, collective karmic force is created. This force keeps individuals moving in the same direction because they think there is nothing else they can do. Maybe they use different terms for their habits and the intentions they relentlessly create. However, in essence, a destructive karmic force carries through us and perpetuates the same old problems on a planetary scale. Another example is the problems with our global environment. On the level of karma, many have not realized that the planet is a living being because they do not acknowledge their own life force. If people could recognize the earth as a living being, then maybe they would act differently toward it.

Many kinds of destructive forces are being unleashed in the world right now. It appears that human beings have a tremendous momentum toward obliterating themselves. They are, in the view of Taoists, on the path toward death, rather than on the path that affirms life.

## WISDOM IS THE CATALYST FOR PEACE

What is the value of growing old? Is there a value to living more years on the face of the earth? From the point of view of joy, how can you age and be more at home within your own body? Now most seventy-five or eighty-five year olds would gladly switch to the physical bodies they had when they were fifteen or twenty. But even if you don't have that body, what can come as you age is a real sense of peace inside yourself, which many call wisdom. This wisdom gives you the potential to see things as they are and to recognize whether courses of action are sensible or infantile, foolish and ultimately destructive or healthy and balanced. Wisdom gives you the power to get out of linear ruts.

If people don't clear out enough of the chi blockages in their karma, however, they never cultivate wisdom. Even if nanotechnology finds a way to enable people to live to be 300 years old and have bodies that work reasonably well, it will not produce people who are wise, who are at peace with themselves and who are willing to do what they can to help promote sanity and peace in the world.

# HEALING THE WORLD

The planet does not need us. We need it. It can be a planet that either supports us as human beings or ushers us on our way toward death and destruction. At this time, the human population is relearning and repeating many lessons. The current state of the world is the result of massive karmic blockages on a cosmic scale. Even the planet itself is now in danger. If we remain on the same path, the planet will likely enact a defense mechanism that will threaten our human existence.

We have reached a state of imbalance in both our internal and external worlds. This massive buildup of karma is reversible, but it requires many individuals to shift away from karmic ruts. Why don't more people choose to release karmic blockages? Because it requires turning inward, connecting with your body, mind and emotions as one unified whole. Eventually you must face and root out your deepest fears and inner demons. You must assume full responsibility for your actions. As we start to work with our karma, cosmic forces come to our aid. It is a great and noble cause that all of us must undertake to become fully conscious beings.

Until you heal your own personal karma, you can't start to heal the karma of the world. You don't have the inner strength to do it. The greatest thing about dealing with the energy of karma is that it leads you inside yourself. You will feel truly stable, have a sense of peace, and overcome spiritual malaise as well as mental and emotional paralysis so that you are willing to effectively extend outside yourself. Just as the Taoists have given us a method for dealing with our own darker natures and restoring our inner balance, they have given us an equally important way to deal with the karma of more destructive forces in the universe. Balance can be restored.

You will be capable of taking action for the betterment of whatever you're able to do—be it in your local community, village, city, country or the world. If millions of individuals start doing something about the energy that has become blocked in their personal karma, then who knows? Things might get a whole lot better. It's a synergy. Enough people could provide a tipping point.

In the modern Western world, people are materially rich but spiritually poor. We live in large homes but have very little space inside our hearts and minds. Quantity is valued more than quality. Life is busy, over-stimulating and out of balance. At its core, the Chi Revolution is about how we can reclaim our inner lives and achieve balance on a planetary scale.

Energy is always moving toward more life or death. It never stays still. In which direction are *you* moving?

# Section Three

## The Chi Rev Workout

CHAPTER
15

# Five Energy Exercises for Life

*Before teaching chi gung and tai chi, I worked for an environmental and consumer activist group, doing seventy to eighty very stressful hours a week. Yet I could maintain my energy over time using the internal energy practices I learned from Bruce Frantzis. Whenever I would feel burnout coming on, I would just practice more.*

—Bill Ryan, Founder, Brookline Tai Chi,
Brookline, Massachusetts, and the Moving Tiger Energy Exercise Method™

The Chi Rev Workout will ignite a powerful transformative process inside your body. Setting aside just fifteen minutes a day will be your first step toward developing internal sensitivity and the mind-body-spirit connection. The main function of the exercises is to begin activating your chi flow—promoting energetic fitness, the foundation for health, joy, longevity and vitality. You can do any portion of the Chi Rev Workout independently when you need a short break to relieve stress or when you just want to rejuvenate yourself. The principles used in the exercises will also energetically enhance your other exercise programs, so integrating them into your other workouts is highly recommended.

## FIVE HIGH-ENERGY, LOW-IMPACT EXERCISES

The Chi Rev Workout consists of five high-energy, low-impact exercises that will help you find out where your chi is blocked and will eventually release any blockages. With practice, the chi in your body will begin to dramatically increase and flow more smoothly. You will be amazed at the impact these exercises have on increasing your energy levels and decreasing your tension.

The first two exercises, Longevity Breathing and Chi Scanning, require little external movement. You can do them sitting, standing or lying down. These techniques are particularly significant because they can be integrated into any exercise system or work activity. The last three movements—Chi Balancing, Heart Opening and Freeing Trapped Chi energy exercises—are derived from an ancient and renowned chi gung (energy work) exercise method from China called Dragon and Tiger medical chi gung. The system, which is 1,500 years old, has withstood the test of time; it can hardly be called a "fad." Dragon and Tiger is based on Chinese acupuncture. Acupuncturists attempt to heal illness and pain by inserting needles into specific energetic pathways to stimulate and balance chi flow throughout the body. Increased energy flow through a damaged area can release chi blockages, thereby improving blood circulation, regenerating damaged tissues and mitigating chronic illness and pain. An increase in chi flow in one pathway will stimulate greater flows in others. Dragon and Tiger trains you to use your hands, breath and simple body movements to accomplish the same energetic balancing as acupuncture.

I learned and practiced this system when I worked in medical clinics in China. In 1990, I began teaching it for the first time in the West. I saw firsthand how this system enhances the natural healing capacities of the body. The simple, effective movements have been used by 15 to 20 million Chinese people to help combat cancer or to mitigate the effects of chemotherapy and radiation. I have taught it to several students who have used it in their own cancer treatments, some of whom are in remission.

# ENERGETIC FITNESS NOURISHED BY MODERATION

The heart of all energy practices is moderation—the seventy percent rule—neither doing too much or too little, discussed in detail in Chapter 4. As with all chi practices, you strive without pushing beyond seventy percent of your natural capacity. Your computer system is most efficient when functioning at well under its total capacity. When the hard drive is almost full and all of the memory is being used, the system will most likely start to malfunction. The same is true for human beings, although we do not often think about or apply this principle to ourselves.

The Taoists found that straining actually does not help people progress faster or further. Instead, it typically depletes our energy and makes us more fatigued, anxious and nervous. Constant pushing and forcing does not allow our nerves and muscles to relax and return to their natural resting state. Your nerves need downtime, which is not always accomplished during sleep. As soon as we strain or go beyond our capacity, our bodies have a tendency to tense up or shut down, making it ever more difficult for us to be consciously aware of what is happening in our bodies. Although it may seem counterintuitive, the more you relax, the more energy, stamina and strength you will gain and the more your range of motion will improve. By staying within your comfort zone, your physical tension and subliminal psychological stress will gradually decrease and, in time, disappear. Your health will improve and with it your baseline mood, so you experience less frustration and anxiety and more playfulness and joy.

In the Chi Rev Workout, incorporating the simple principle of the seventy percent rule will help you achieve all the physical and energetic benefits faster. It will help improve how deeply you breathe, how much time you practice, how much mental or physical energy you expend and how much you stretch or bend your arms, legs or torso.

If you are injured or ill with any kind of chronic condition, or you have a cold or flu, you should temporarily practice the Chi Rev Workout using the forty or fifty percent rule until you are healed. This may include doing movements while sitting or lying down. Once you are healed, you can resume practice to seventy percent of your capacity. By embracing this rule, you will develop an internal chi sensor that allows you to gauge your energy level at any given time. It will further signal you to either slow down or pick up the pace. Over time, you will be able to observe those around you in a similar manner for effective communication. This is a particularly useful tool when leading groups, teaching or parenting.

The next section gives a quick overview of the five exercises so you'll be ready to practice them when they are detailed in subsequent chapters.

# THE SET

## Energy Exercise 1: Longevity Breathing

The first exercise of the Chi Rev Workout is based on Longevity Breathing—an advanced breathing system I developed from ancient Taoist techniques. Practicing will continually and dramatically increase your energy and vitality. Longevity Breathing is a powerful technique to become conscious of the inside of your physical body and its energies. Breath training helps you make the link between breathing patterns and your chi. Eventually you will create a positive feedback loop. Eastern and Western medical practitioners have long recognized the value of the breath to improve health and release tension. Many alternative healers and therapists teach breathing exercises as a fundamental practice to help their clients relax. Breathing well helps athletes of any sport to improve their concentration and focus while maintaining a high level of energy to stay "in the zone."

Breath training is part of most energy exercise systems, such as tai chi, chi gung and TAO yoga because awareness and strength of the breath helps people feel and increase their chi. Breathing techniques are also found in other exercise programs such as weightlifting and Pilates. Not surprising, breath training provides the foundation for many spiritual traditions, such as Buddhism, where breathing becomes the path to quiet the monkey mind and center one's attention for long periods.

## Energy Exercise 2: Chi Scanning

Chi Scanning is the introductory practice for helping you recognize where chi is blocked in your body. You'll need to know how to locate blockages if you wish to do more advanced chi practices that teach you to release blockages. These methods were passed down by Lao Tse, author of the *Tao Te Ching,* over 2,500 years ago. Chi Scanning is also one of the foundation practices for developing the power of your intention, which can be directed outward, toward any goal, or inward, toward more advanced meditation work and/or prayer.

## Energy Exercise 3: Chi Balancing

The next three exercises, which are part of Dragon and Tiger chi gung, wake up your chi and get it going. Your breath, hand movements and intention are used to strongly increase and balance your chi, get rid of blocked chi and help you put your attention on such positive emotions as love and compassion.

The Chi Balancing energy exercise gives you a general energetic tune-up and clears the mind and emotions for inner stability. You get the chi going by balancing and increasing the flow of chi along two of the three main chi superhighways inside your body. Your hand movements will strongly and positively activate and heal the energy of the liver and lungs as you move them along the same meridian lines used in acupuncture. This is a great exercise to do after you've been sitting at your computer for a while, when you feel yourself getting uptight or in a bad mood or when you feel drained and sleepy.

## Energy Exercise 4: Heart Opening

The Heart Opening exercise benefits your physical heart, helping you to open to compassion and love. Your heart is not just the key to your body's circulation and wellness; it is the seat of your consciousness and awareness. On a physical level, this exercise helps improve blood circulation while clearing the heart and its arteries of chi blockages. On a metaphysical level, this movement affects the heart tantien or chakra, which is located in the central chi superhighway. It develops your ability to strongly send out and receive compassion and love. Spiritually, it helps open your heart and trains you to consciously use your intention to go outside of yourself for the sake of others. It will help you counter the natural "What's in it for me?" voice in your head.

## Energy Exercise 5: Freeing Trapped Chi

The Freeing Trapped Chi exercise helps you to relax and let go. Many people clutch at life rather than relaxing into it. I wrote an entire book devoted to the subject of meditation, *Relaxing Into Your Being,* to help my students make the shift from a stress response to a relaxation response. Human beings commonly hold on to control rather than let go. Burdens prevent us from becoming fully alive and joyful. Have you ever watched a cat or dog after a confrontation? They typically shake it all off, literally. This is part of the process of releasing what has become stuck inside them so they can continue with their lazy day. This potent exercise gradually helps you release and let go of the small historical shocks and emotional residues you have accumulated in your life. It is equally powerful for releasing larger shocks and traumas. The personal experience of emotional pain, such as anger, sadness or fear, or the inner trauma that occurs after a serious shock such as an earthquake, hurricane or car accident makes it very difficult to focus on virtually anything else. You will learn to release shocks out of your system, calm yourself down and enable your body to begin the healing process.

# ESTABLISHING A PRACTICE ROUTINE

The best way to incorporate a new habit and rhythm into your life is to set aside a particular time and place to do it. Here are a few suggestions for when to practice the Chi Rev Workout:

- Early morning before you get distracted.
- Before or after other exercises that you regularly do, such as walking, biking, running or working out at your gym.
- When you return home from work and need to cool down, or if you need to take a break during work.

Once you've figured out a place and time, make a commitment of fifteen minutes. You could start with five minutes and work up to ten or fifteen. If you start with five minutes, pick only one of the Chi Rev Workout exercises to learn and practice that day; move onto the next only when you are ready.

# NOURISHING YOUR INNER REVOLUTION

Practicing the Chi Rev Workout will help you create your own inner revolution. You are shifting your attention inward so you can develop consciousness inside yourself and get your chi going. As you practice the Chi Rev Workout, you might gradually begin noticing that some of the discomforts you used to feel are relieved or disappear altogether, indicating that these exercises are working for you.

# CHAPTER 16

# Longevity Breathing

When a hundred or so students signed up for my Longevity Breathing retreat in Crete, many of the Greeks thought the whole thing was nuts. "Look at those crazy people. They spent all that money on learning to do what we do naturally every day!" If there were only one thing I could do to help Westerners, it would be to teach them to breathe well. If you do nothing else except learn to breathe well, it will dramatically improve the quality of your life. Learning to breathe properly is one of the most important portals to healing, relaxation, rejuvenating sleep, athletics, martial arts, graceful aging and spirituality.

## SHALLOW BREATHING

Doctors report that up to ninety percent of Americans do not fully use their diaphragms while breathing. They take shallow breaths and only use a portion of the lungs, even when they believe they are taking deep breaths. Not using the rest of the lungs is like starving the body from one of its most important rejuvenators. Holding the breath is particularly common when people are angry and fearful, tense or highly focused; it often results in the nervous system reacting to the pressure with a physiologically based stress response. When you contract, your chi is inherently blocked from moving freely and locks up somewhere in the body, most commonly the shoulders, stomach or jaw. Moreover, when people take shallower and shallower breaths or hold their breath, their bodies become more and more sluggish. Releasing stress becomes difficult so tension lodges in the body and cells. Over time, it takes progressively more energy to maintain the same amount of concentration or physical activity. Imagine what happens to your body as you age.

In one of my stress-reduction seminars, I asked business executives to type lecture notes on their laptop computers while *simultaneously* remaining aware of their breath. Within minutes, most of the participants' breath became shallower. Many of them stopped breathing for seconds at a time. Many were lucky if out of a minute, they actually breathed continuously for ten seconds. Executives, many of whom are high-functioning and extremely intelligent individuals, were surprised to learn they had such a difficult time maintaining the smooth flow of breath while working on their computers.

## REJUVENATING BENEFITS

I frequently ask my students, "What is breathing?" The standard reply is that air comes in and out of the nose, thereby pumping more oxygen into the body. Although technically true, the story is incomplete. There are several main reasons why shallow breathers should learn Longevity Breathing:

- o To fully engage the diaphragm, which physically causes air to enter and leave the lungs.
- o To recondition the nervous system from the reflex of perpetually going into stress to the reflex of normally going into relaxation.
- o To improve the circulation of fluids and the natural movement within the internal organs, making them less prone to disease.

- To help the body rest and receive the optimal benefits of sleep.
- To deliver more oxygen to all of the cells.
- To strengthen the movement of chi.

My Longevity Breathing program, developed from Taoist practices, can make the inside of your body fully alive and healthy. It cultivates your ability to relax at any time and to concentrate on what you are doing for long periods without becoming distracted. It gets your chi going. Breathing properly is key to a healing, restful night's sleep. When you are stressed out, even after you fall asleep, it takes some hours for the nerves to fully release. The nerves must be relaxed before they can start the repair process. Moreover, when the nerves have shut down from stress, less oxygen circulates throughout the body. Lessening the recovery time and increasing oxygenation in the brain will help you to let go once you fall asleep faster.

*I was diagnosed with emphysema in 1994. Like many people, I was a shallow breather. Taoist breathing taught me how to exercise unused portions of my lungs and strengthen them. In 2000, a lung function test showed an increase from 17% to 47%.*

Walter Rapaport, Recording Engineer, Jerome, Arizona

## TRAINING FOR RELAXATION

Longevity Breathing helps open up your body and counter the involuntary clench of tension with relaxation. Of course, it takes training to recognize the connection between your breath and your emotions, particularly when the negative emotions come crashing in. Most have never considered that they are capable of keeping their composure even in stressful situations. However, as you practice Longevity Breathing, you learn to use this important skill to calm yourself down, helping you to act with clarity, so you don't make a negative event worse. The calmer you are, the more easily your chi flows and grows. The steadier and less inhibited the chi flow, the more oxygen the cells can absorb. As your cells receive reinforcement—continuous breathing over weeks, months and years—they become more efficient, improving your circulation. It is a powerful synergy. Most people have trained their bodies to be tense and hard, which in turn restricts their chi flow. Longevity Breathing will train you to become relaxed and a little looser.[1] Creating stable, ongoing, continuous relaxation cannot occur from a place of tension. Some may be able to create a short-lived sense of relaxation from tension, but not a sense of ongoing well-being that fills you up with chi, your life force.

## Longevity Breathing Begins with Belly Breathing

The basic nature of Longevity Breathing is to get everything inside your body—muscles, internal organs, fluids—to move in sync with your breathing. Belly breathing creates one rhythm using the metronome of your breath, patterned after that of babies. Everything inside a baby's body moves in tandem with his or her breath, the secret to the infant's boundless, virtually limitless energy. When you breathe from your belly, you pressurize the inside of your stomach cavity—front, sides and back—thereby moving your diaphragm and drawing air into the entirety of your lungs. As your lungs fill with air, all your internal organs, tissues and blood vessels expand. Instead of feeling sluggish or contracted, this kind of breathing fully wakes you up, increases your ability to focus and gives you more energy without the buzzing sensation associated with caffeine intake or an adrenaline rush.

## MASSAGING YOUR INTERNAL ORGANS

Breathing with the belly moves the diaphragm strongly, as is commonly found in many breathing systems. What is unique to this system, however, is that the beginning stage of belly breathing

[1] You can learn Longevity Breathing principles in more detail in the author's book, *Opening the Energy Gates of Your Body* or from his *Longevity Breathing* DVD and *Taoist Breathing* CD.

as well as the later stages of Longevity Breathing, very gently massage your internal organs—liver, spleen, kidneys and the back of the heart. Gentle massaging is all that is necessary to improve blood circulation and lengthen connections between tendons and ligaments.

Although many of us know the importance of exercising our muscles, the idea of exercising the internal organs is something we may have never considered. Illnesses rarely present themselves in the strongest parts of the body. But, as with any system, you are only as strong as your weakest link. What are some of the scariest illnesses? Those that attack our internal organs—our liver, kidneys, spleen, lungs, intestines, heart. Over time and without exercise, the internal motion inside the organs slows down and diminishes the flow of blood and other fluids within them. The connecting ligaments and tendons respond by contracting, bringing the organs closer together and limiting mobility and circulation. Eventually, they harden and complications arise. Using the breath to strengthen the internal organs is a big deal, not a small one. It will help you to stay healthy.

## INCREASE YOUR MENTAL STAMINA

In Western culture, one image that seems to exemplify people in deep concentration is the sculpture by Rodin called *The Thinker.* Here is a guy sitting there, appearing to say to himself, "I'm going to figure this out—or else." Basically, he is hunched over and punching himself in the jaw—not exactly a poster child for relaxation. How long do you think that thinker could hold this position? Maybe ten or fifteen minutes? Probably not for three hours.

Now consider the figure of the Buddha sitting quietly and serenely while he is in contemplation. He could easily sit there for a week. And many experienced meditators do sit for weeks at a time. When you are relaxed, your concentration and focus have immense stamina. Conversely, tension eats stamina. Although it may seem counterintuitive at first, relaxation increases strength and stamina. Relaxed breathing nourishes and increases mental stamina.

## LONGEVITY BREATHING EXERCISES

These easy exercises will help you begin the process of breathing smoothly, evenly and strongly while developing your ability to stay focused. You might consider consciously setting aside five minutes in the Chi Rev Workout for practicing Longevity Breathing. Although it is easiest to learn these breathing exercises as part of the Chi Rev Workout, they can be practiced anytime—just after waking up or before falling asleep, on the bus, taxi, plane or subway, during work, etc.—and in any position—standing, sitting or lying down.

Lying on your back is the simplest position for learning these exercises. You can stretch out your legs or raise your knees, whichever makes you feel more comfortable. You can also sit in a chair, as long as you gently lift and straighten your spine and do not allow it to slump.

Although these exercises are very easy, some of my students report that they find breathing exercises a little on the boring side. In this situation, I have found that TAO yoga, discussed in Chapter 10, is particularly useful as a vehicle for these students to practice their breathing exercises. They can move a little bit and open up their bodies with the gentle postures to get the chi going while keeping their monkey minds focused.

### Basic Principles
As you do any of the following breathing exercises, you may find it helpful to follow a few principles:

- Breathe softly; no forcing or pushing is necessary.
- Breathe through your nose unless you have specific medical problems that prevent you from doing so.
- Do not strain by trying to take a longer breath or forcing the breath in any way whatsoever; moderation—the seventy percent rule—is paramount.

○ Keep your tongue on the roof of your mouth and as relaxed as you can; this contact connects two major chi flows in the body.

## Feel Your Breath: One Minute

Breathe in and breathe out. Focus on taking a measure of what your breath feels like. Before you can change anything or learn new ways of breathing, you need to take stock of where you are right now. Don't be concerned with trying to change anything. Ask yourself, "What are some of the qualities of my breath?" Do not focus on interpretations. Human beings naturally analyze; just gently guide your attention back to the inhale-exhale. Here are some things to gently focus on:

○ Is your inhale longer than your exhale or vice versa?
○ Do you involuntarily hold your breath between the inhale-exhale and, vice versa, between the exhale-inhale?
○ As you inhale or exhale, are there places where your breath seems to spurt or jerk?
○ Is your breathing relaxed or tense? Do you have to maintain strain or effort to breathe?

Give it a go now.

## Use Your Breath to Consciously Relax: One Minute

Use your conscious intention to just start relaxing your body in coordination with your breath. Very deliberately, as your breath comes in, relax. As your breath goes out, let go and relax more. This will help you begin to associate the act of breathing with relaxing your body. Put your attention on your face, neck and shoulders, a place where many hold tension. Is the inhale or exhale making you tenser, or more relaxed? Just notice what is really going on as you breathe and forget why.

Once you discover the level of tension that is working in you right now, every time you inhale and exhale, deliberately relax those places in your body that involuntarily tense without you telling them to do so. Just bringing some conscious attention to places that are commonly tensed as you breathe will help gently relax them. You will find that if you let your breath be steady and soft, the tension will more easily release. If you tense your muscles, your breath gets choppy—having a start-and-stop, start-and-stop, start-and-stop quality. You will probably notice that when there is a sense of tension in your breathing, your muscles cannot relax. They will either maintain their level of tension or get even tenser. Try to breathe as softly, steadily and calmly as you can. With each breath, see if can let your tension go a little more—if you can. If not, it's okay. In time, you will.

Take a minute now.

## Breathe without Holding the Breath: One Minute

Many people hold their breath between the inhale and exhale or vice versa, particularly when they are highly focused, tense, excited, frightened or angry. Habitually holding the breath creates tension in the nervous system. So, next, focus on making your breath smooth between the inhale-exhale and vice versa, without stops and starts.

You know what to do...

## Breathe with Your Belly: Two Minutes

Put one hand on your belly and one hand on your chest. Gently push your belly so that it sticks out to inhale and draw in air. When you exhale, relax and allow your belly to return to its original position. Two points to remember:

○ The front of your chest should stay still and be relaxed, moving neither up nor down, forward nor backward; see if you can let all your inhales and exhales come directly from the movement of your belly.
○ Don't be concerned with the length of your breath; however, see if you can make each inhale and exhale approximately the same length.

# BUILDING A LIFE-SUSTAINING FOUNDATION

This introduction to Longevity Breathing provides you with the
basics of one of the most powerful methods ever developed for
increasing your energy and vitality while decreasing stress and
anxiety. These simple exercises help you tune into your physical
body and the energies that run your thoughts and emotions.
Longevity Breathing teaches you to become aware of how your chi
is affected by your breath, to calm your monkey mind and keep
your focus—the foundation of all chi practices.

We all know that we have internal organs, but most of us do not
consider that the quality of our lives is determined by the quality of
the internal function of our bodies. I wonder what in life you would
think is worth having if you didn't have your health to enjoy it.

CHAPTER 17

# Chi Scanning

You need not go to the Himalayas to explore and become inspired. There is a hidden ecology beneath your own skin, which can spring to life, flourish and grow as you put your mind deeper and deeper into the uncharted wilderness of your own body. Chi Scanning is a foundation step in tuning into your body's inner ecology. This powerful exercise asks you to stand, turn inward and systematically scan inside your body from the top of your head to the bottom of your feet. Through this process, you will become reacquainted with the inside of your body so you can recognize where tension resides and forms chi blockages. Your tools to feel these blockages are your awareness, attention and intention.

The ability to feel inside your body allows you to continuously monitor whether your systems are optimal, normal or downgraded. Many people don't discover that they have serious health issues until the condition has advanced because they don't feel the subtle onset of symptoms or changes inside their bodies during the early stages. Once you can feel inside your body, you will begin to differentiate between optimal, normal and downgraded.

# Relaxing the Monkey Mind

Most people can't focus on only one subject at a time because their minds jump from one subject to another like a monkey swinging from tree to tree. Their minds juggle their "to do" lists; headaches or other pains; worries about their jobs, children, or parents; the fight they had with their husbands, wives, superiors. The Taoists call this kind of thinking the "10,000 agendas," which is actually just a metaphor since it might be possible to conceive of many more agendas.

By focusing inwards, Chi Scanning provides the opportunity to observe how active your monkey mind is and calm it down. Chi Scanning is not about focusing on your thoughts. It is about getting into your body and *feeling* how your thoughts affect your body. You won't be able to resolve anything with your thoughts, although your mind will have you *think* it is possible. Chi Scanning helps calm the monkey mind because it brings your chi from your head down to your feet. One of my students told me that when she has insomnia, she does Chi Scanning in bed; most of the time, she falls asleep before reaching her feet.

As you scan, give yourself permission to set aside the 10,000 agendas for a few minutes—they might not completely go away, but in those few moments, you give them a chance to relax. Perhaps when you go back to them, they might be calmer or, better yet, hardly there at all.

## Start with Good Posture

The way you stand has a great deal to do with whether your chi flows smoothly in your body or gets kinked and blocked much like a plumbing system. Water flows less smoothly in places where the pipes form a U-joint or where they have become clogged with gunk. Similarly, chi will not flow smoothly when your normal posture is hunched over, when you stand rigidly on one leg, when your stomach is clenched, your legs are crossed or your shoulders are hunched up near your ears. Smooth out the plumbing, and you'll get better flow and allow your chi to grow. Chi Scanning is commonly done standing. However, if you can't stand because of any pain or illness, then you can do this exercise sitting or lying down.

## Six Fundamental Principles

There are six fundamentals to standing well, but if you cannot fulfill all of them while staying relaxed and comfortable, don't fret. Most people can't easily fulfill most of the requirements because of poor postural habits acquired from childhood and from leaning toward computer screens—just look at Bill Gates! As you practice, your body will slowly relax and these checkpoints will become easier to maintain:

- Your feet are parallel, shoulder's width apart.
- Your weight is evenly balanced on both feet.
- No joints are locked; your knees are slightly bent.
- Your muscles are relaxed, not clenched, particularly the jaw, stomach and buttocks muscles.
- Your shoulders are relaxed and down.
- Your lower back is straight, perpendicular to the ground, with your head neither tilted forward nor backward.

In advanced chi practices, for optimum chi flow, the checkpoints become stricter and precise alignments are paramount. My *Opening the Energy Gates of Your Body* book covers these alignments in great detail if you prefer more guidance.

## Ready, Set, Scan!

In this chi gung practice, you will internally scan your body from the top of the head down. Your tongue will lightly touch the roof of your mouth to keep two major chi junctions connected. As you scan down, start to notice places in your body where you feel any sense of tension, strength, contraction or any type of binding, especially if you don't know what it is—in other words, any one of the four blockage conditions discussed in Chapter 12. As you explore, simply take inventory of what you feel, noticing any spots—no matter how small or subtle—that reflect any of the four blockage conditions. Do you notice places in your body where you also feel an increase in such negative emotions as anger, fear or sadness? You need not do anything with these sensations: Simply become aware, take inventory of where they are located in your body and forget *why*.

The following is a practical sequence I often give my students to help keep their minds focused. I suggest staying at each spot in the string for two to five breaths since many of these locations are important junctions in your chi highways. Starting at the middle of the top of your head (where the soft spot is in a baby), scan downward to:

The middle of your forehead
Your temples, just above and to the outside side of your eyes
Just behind the center of your eyes and optic nerve
The soft spot just below the ears
The place where your tongue touches the roof of your mouth
Your jaw
Your throat
The top of your shoulders
The inside of your armpits
Your shoulder blades
The front of your breasts or "pecs"
Your ribs
Your stomach
Your buttocks
Your thighs
Your knees
Your ankles
Your feet, and out through your toes.

# STEADY PROGRESSION

What is important as you do this simple scan is to feel rather than visualize. Many people mistakenly think it is enough to visualize these internal spots, which is an infinitely easier task than feeling them. You can imagine and visualize being a duck all you want; but at the end of the day, if you can't lay an egg, you know you're not a duck. The function of standing is to develop the capacity to feel inside your body. Remember to be gentle with yourself and let this be one area of your life where you do not use force.

The process of developing our capacity to feel inside our bodies is gradual and incremental. Only the rarest of human beings can initially do this exercise correctly and maintain awareness throughout the scan for more than a minute or two. As with all chi energy practices, the more gentle and consistent you are with your practice, the more steady your progress.

CHAPTER
18

# Chi Balancing

A key way that you work with your chi in the Chi Balancing exercise is by moving your hands through the chi field that surrounds your body. Your hand movements cause chi to circulate through some of the main acupuncture channels that are located within your body. This works because the chi within your body and the chi in the field outside your body are interconnected. Movement of chi outside causes chi to move inside, and vice versa.

The Chi Balancing exercise is taught in five steps. Each step will incorporate previous steps, building on what you have already mastered. As you are learning, take whatever time you have in your Chi Rev Workout for this exercise and split that time in two parts. During the first part, practice the steps that you have already learned. Devote the second part to learning the next step.

Take your time when learning a new step. Only move on to learn a new step when you feel very comfortable with what you've been practicing. As one of my teachers used to say, "It is better to do one thing well, than many things poorly."

When you have completed all the steps, you will have learned the entire exercise, which you can then just practice in its entirety.

## Step 1. Balance the Chi of Your Legs and Feet

In this step you will learn to move your feet and legs so energy will:

**1.** Rise from the earth into the ball of your foot, and then

**2.** Sink from your heel back to the earth. We naturally exchange chi with the earth through our movements, and the earth can be a great source of chi for us. The movements you will learn in this step will increase the amount of energy you are able to gather from the earth.

In addition, you will begin to balance the amount of chi you have in your legs and feet.

**Beginning position:** *The standing posture you learned in the Chi Scanning exercise (p.159)—face forward, feet flat on the floor, parallel to each other, approximately shoulder's width apart, with your weight distributed evenly on both feet.*

Your goal is to shift your weight back and forth from one foot to the other in a smooth, relaxed manner, and, as you do so, lift and lower the heel of the unweighted foot. When done correctly, you will feel like you are pumping your legs up and down as if riding a bicycle.

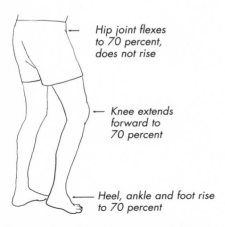

Hip joint flexes to 70 percent, does not rise

Knee extends forward to 70 percent

Heel, ankle and foot rise to 70 percent

*Shift Weight to One Foot and Then the Other*
*1A*

**1.** Shift your body's weight to one foot, keeping your weighted knee slightly bent. Gently exert pressure through that heel. This will cause energy to drop down that side of your body. As you do so, move your other knee forward to slightly lift your heel, while keeping the ball of your foot on the ground. This will cause energy to rise on that side of your body *(Figure 1A).*

**2.** Smoothly lower your heel and shift your weight back to be evenly distributed on both feet.

**3.** Repeat Instruction 1 but shift your body's weight to the other foot, while you move the knee of the unweighted leg forward to raise your heel *(Figure 1B)*.

**4.** Smoothly lower your heel and shift back to the beginning position.

**5.** Repeat Instructions 1 through 4 over and over for as much time as you have in your Chi Rev Workout.

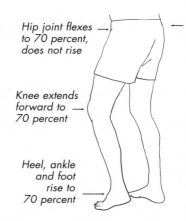

*Hip joint flexes → to 70 percent, does not rise*

*Knee extends forward to → 70 percent*

*Heel, ankle and foot rise to 70 percent*

*Shift Weight to One Foot and Then the Other*
*1B*

Some points to remember as you shift weight:

○ Both of your legs and feet must stay relaxed.

○ Your hips must remain even and not tilted. Try not to shift your hip up or out to the side when you shift weight.

○ Remember the seventy percent rule and lift your heel only as high as you are able to maintain your balance, keep your leg relaxed and stay comfortable.

○ Only shift as much weight as is comfortable. If you need to, allow some weight to remain on your unweighted leg.

As you shift weight, while lifting and lowering your legs and feet, let your movements become very smooth, steady, rhythmical and continuous. Play with finding a slow, steady rhythm that is relaxing and feels good. Move as if you were a big cat, steadily, carefully and consciously. Let all the muscles of your legs, feet and hips relax, so that you use only those muscles necessary for the movement. This will allow your feet to exchange chi with the earth. Try to be aware of every joint in your toes, feet, ankles, knees and hips attempting to move every part in unison in a liquid manner.

Especially emphasize the action of lowering and then putting weight and gentle pressure through each heel. This action causes your chi to drop into the earth through your heel, which in turn causes chi to rise back up your other leg from the earth. When you have mastered this action, you will feel as if the lowering of one heel causes the other heel to rise.

As you play with this movement, let the feelings—and the chi—in your feet, legs and hips come into balance. If you notice that one foot or leg feels more alive and liquid than the other, put a little more of your attention into the less alive foot or leg so that you awaken it and bring more chi to it. Be aware of what feels good about the more alive foot or leg. Experiment with how you can change the way you do the movement so that both feet and legs start to feel equally alive and balanced.

## STEP 2. BRING CHI UP AND DOWN ONE LEG WITH ONE HAND

In this step you will learn to move your hands through your energy field to cause energy to:

**1.** Rise from the earth up the inside of your leg, the front of your hip and then up the torso to the front of your shoulder, and

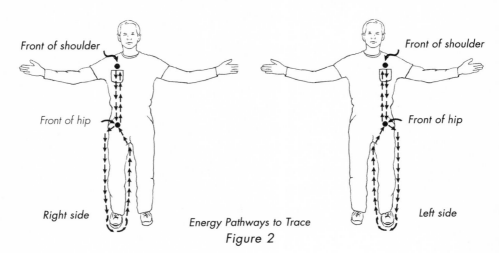

Energy Pathways to Trace
Figure 2

**2.** Sink back down the front of your torso to the front of your hip, around it and down the outside of your leg to the earth.

The energy pathways your hands will trace are shown in *Figure 2.* The movements you will learn in this step will increase the amount of chi you exchange with the earth and will increase the amount of chi you have in your body.

## Upward Movement

Choose one hand with which to learn this step first. When you become comfortable with one hand, then try it with the other.

Keep your hand 6–8 inches away from your body at all times.

**Beginning position:** *Feet parallel, shoulder's width apart with your weight evenly distributed on both feet. Your arms rest comfortably at your sides, with your armpits slightly open. Your fingers point downwards at the outsides of your feet (Figure 3A).*

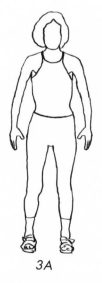

3A

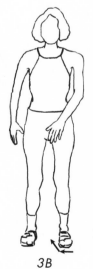

*Keep your arm loose and relaxed as you circle your arm inward around your foot. Your palm will face the inside of your leg*

3B

**1.** Choose which hand and arm you want to use. Circle that arm forward and inward around your foot so that your fingers first point at the tips of your toes and then at the inside of your foot *(Figure 3B).*

2. Slowly pull your arm up and with your hand trace the energy pathways from your foot along the inside of your knee and thigh to the front of your hip. Imagine you are pulling energy up the inside of your leg *(Figure 3C)*.

3. When your hand reaches the front of your hip, gradually turn your palm to face upwards as you bring your hand up the front of your torso to your nipple and then to the front of your shoulder *(Figure 3D)*.

Try to let your elbow stay relaxed and feel slightly heavy, and keep your shoulders down.

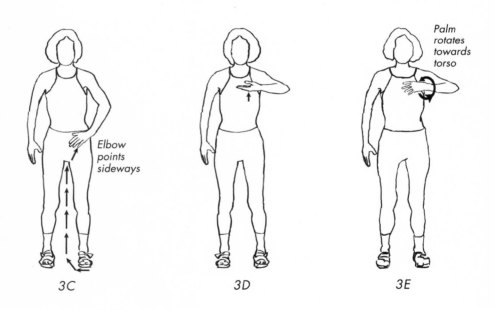

*Elbow points sideways*

*Palm rotates towards torso*

3C                          3D                          3E

## Downward Movement

4. At the top of your upward hand movement, turn your palm over so that it faces the ground *(Figure 3E)*.

**5.** In a relaxed way, push your palm down to your nipple and then to the front of your hip *(Figure 3F)*.

**6.** Move your palm around to face the outside of your hip *(Figure 3G)*.

**7.** Lower your palm slowly down the outside of your leg until  your fingertips face toward the outside of your foot *(Figure 3H)*. Try not to reach so far that you lock your arm. As you do this, your palm will face towards your thigh. While your hand falls, imagine you are pushing energy down the outside of your leg to the outside of your foot.

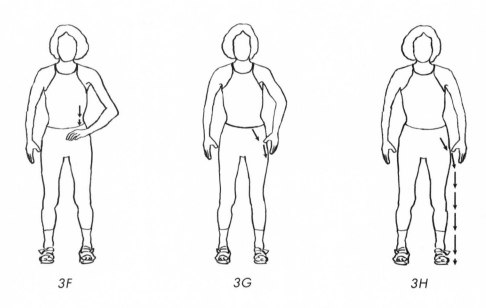

*3F*                              *3G*                              *3H*

## Repeat Up and Down Movements

Repeat the upward and downward movements until you feel competent without having to refer to this text or illustrations. Your goal is to practice until you can trace the correct energy pathways in a smooth, relaxed motion on both sides of your body.

As you move your arm up and down, feel as if you are gently pushing your hand through water. Try to maintain this feeling in your hand at all times as you move it up and down. Sometimes, the movements of tai chi and chi gung are called "swimming on dry land" because practitioners strive to maintain this feeling.

When you feel you can trace the energy pathways in a smooth relaxed motion, begin using the other hand.

## How High Do I Raise My Palm?

Initially, the ideal height is in front of your collarbone. This is the optimal height for physically loosening your shoulder.

However, when you begin learning this movement, it may only feel comfortable to raise your hand as high as the bottom of your ribs. With practice you will gradually reach the nipple, the front of your shoulder and then the collarbone. If you are stiff or injured, only raise your hand to a height that does not cause tension or pain to begin. The highest you should raise your hands is to your collarbone. Although you may be physically able to raise your hands higher, you will not gain any energetic benefit by doing so.

Energetically, the ideal height is just a little lower than the collarbone in front of the shoulder, that is after you are stretched and can comfortably reach your collarbone. There you will have the strongest positive effect on stimulating energy flows in this area.

By staying within your comfort boundary as you repeat the movements, your physical tension will gradually decrease and in time disappear. It may take you a few weeks or months to get your hands all the way to your collarbone, but when you do, your energy will flow more strongly than if you had forced your shoulders to stretch.

## STEP 3. COORDINATE RAISING AND LOWERING ONE HAND AND HEEL

Your goal is to lift and lower your hand and heel on one side of your body in unison. Ideally, your hand and heel begin to move and finish moving upward or downward at the same time. This is challenging because the tendency of many people is to have the heel rise and fall faster than the hand.

As in the previous step, choose one hand with which to learn this step first. When you become comfortable with that hand, then try it with the other hand.

Keep your hand 6–8 inches away from your body at all times.

**Beginning position:** *Feet flat on the floor, parallel to each other, approximately shoulder's width apart. The weight is distributed evenly on both feet. Place both hands comfortably at your sides, open your armpits slightly and point your left fingers at the outside of your left foot (Figure 4A).*

1. Choose which hand and foot you wish to use. Circle your arm forward so that your fingers point at the tips of your toes and then at the inside of your foot *(Figure 4B)*.
2. On the same side as that arm, begin to shift your weight and raise your heel. With your palm trace the energy pathways up the inside of your leg to the front of your hip *(Figure 4C)*. At this point, your heel will be raised halfway.

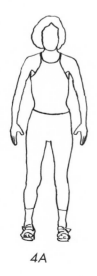

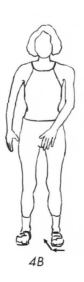

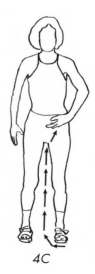

*4A*                    *4B*                    *4C*

3. Finish shifting your weight and raise your heel to its maximum comfortable height as you turn your palm upward and bring it to the front of your shoulder *(Figure 4D)*.

4. Rotate your palm to face down, begin lowering your heel, and move your palm down to the front and then side of your hip *(Figure 4E–G)*. At this point, your heel will be lowered halfway.

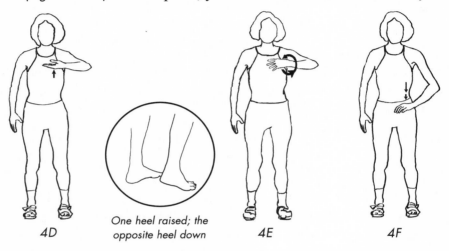

4D          *One heel raised; the opposite heel down*          4E          4F

5. When your hand has finished tracing the energy pathways down to your foot, your heel will be fully lowered. Shift your weight to be distributed evenly on both feet *(Figure 4G-H)*.

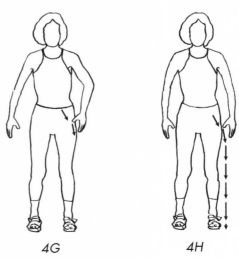

4G                    4H

Practice coordinating the timing of your hand and heel rising and falling a minimum of twenty times.

When you are comfortable with working on one side, you can then learn to smoothly raise and lower your opposite hand and heel.

## STEP 4. THE WHOLE EXERCISE

Now you are ready to put the whole movement together.

There is no need to be concerned about learning the movement perfectly. Doing it more or less correctly is quite acceptable. Be gentle with yourself and do not try to be perfect.

**Beginning position:** *Stand comfortably, feet parallel, shoulder's width apart, with your weight evenly distributed on both feet. Your arms rest comfortably at your sides, palms facing the outsides of legs and fingers pointing toward the floor. Maintain a little space within both armpits and keep your elbows slightly bent (Figure 5A).*

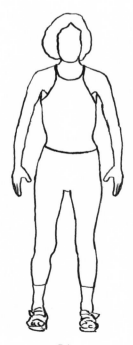

5A

Breathe comfortably using the techniques of the Longevity Breathing exercise. Let your breath become very steady and relaxed. Let your mind become calm and feel your breath move in and out of your body. Let your thoughts drop away and prepare to begin the movement.

## Preparation

The exercise begins by moving one hand and foot only. You have already learned these movements previously.

**1.** Choose a hand and heel to move first. Circle that arm forward and in so that your fingers point at the inside of your foot, begin to shift your weight to your other foot and slightly raise your heel *(Figure 5B)*.

**2.** Trace the energy pathways up to the front of your hip *(Figure 5C)*. Raise your heel halfway.

**3.** Finish shifting your weight, raise your heel to seventy percent of its maximum comfortable height, gradually turn your palm upward and bring it up to the front of your shoulder *(Figure 5D)*.

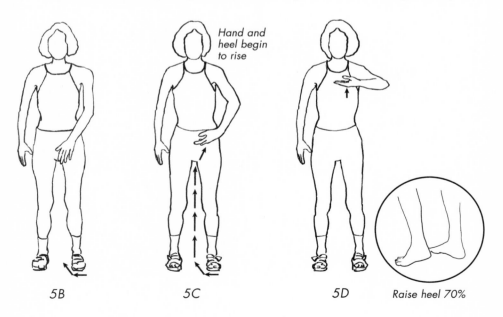

Hand and heel begin to rise

5B          5C          5D          *Raise heel 70%*

You are now ready to begin coordinating the hands and feet on both sides.

## PUTTING IT ALL TOGETHER

1. As you circle your lower arm forward and inward, rotate your upper palm down *(Figure 5E)*.

2. As the upper hand and heel on the same side of your body begin to move downwards, your lower hand and heel begin to rise. The hands should pass each other at the front of the hip. Ideally, both heels are just slightly off the ground as the hands pass each other. At this point, however, your falling heel can touch the ground sooner if that makes it easier to keep your balance *(Figure 5F)*.

3. Shift your weight as you move your falling hand around your hip and down your leg, your rising hand up to the front of your shoulder, and your heel as high as is comfortable *(Figure 5G)*.

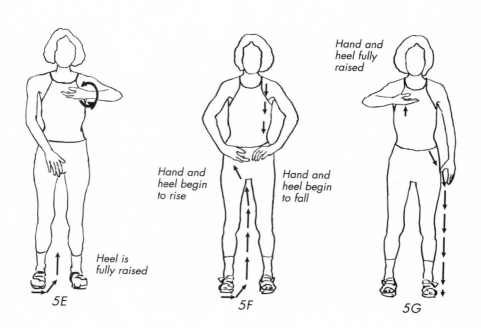

Hand and heel fully raised

Hand and heel begin to rise

Hand and heel begin to fall

Heel is fully raised

5E

5F

5G

Repeat Instructions 1-3 in a continuous loop *(Figure 5E–G to 5H–J)*, with one hand and heel moving up while the opposite hand and heel goes down.

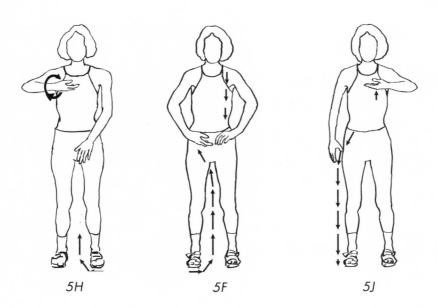

5H                         5F                         5J

When you first begin practing this step, pause for a moment each time that you have one hand fully up and one hand fully down. Relax, breathe a few times, and adjust as necessary to get your arms, hands, legs and feet into their desired positions. Try to do these moves without any strain, muscular strength or tension anywhere in your body; if you do feel these qualities, try to relax and release them. The goal is to try to have all parts of your body feel relatively springy, alive and fully relaxed.

When you have practiced this step for a while and become comfortable with all the positions and the timing, then leave out any pauses and begin to smoothly shift from up to down and right to left, and vice versa. Eventually you will want your movements to become continuous, steady, and rhythmical.

Practice this step until you can do the movements fairly well without having to think about them.

# STEP 5. USE THE EXERCISE TO BALANCE YOUR CHI

Now you can start to use the exercise to balance the chi of your feet, legs, hands, arms and torso.

Begin to do the exercise slowly, steadily, and continuously. Try to keep your arms and hands and your legs and feet moving at all times. If you stop moving a part of your body for an instant, then your chi circulation in that part of your body will slow or even stop. It will lag behind the circulation in other parts of your body and your overall chi flow will become less balanced. So the first step in balancing your chi is to move continuously.

The next step is to notice which parts of your body feel more alive and easy to move and which feel less responsive and more sluggish or tight. For a while just practice feeling your body as you do the movements. Be aware of what you notice, but do not try to do anything yet. Relax and open your mind and let yourself learn to feel many parts of your body simultaneously.

Once you can do this a bit, then begin to play within your body. Put a little more attention into the parts of your body which feel less alive and responsive. Play with how you do the movements so that you try to awaken these areas. For example, you might exaggerate how you move those areas or how you move your hands across those areas to make them more alive.

## Moving with the Breath

You can also use your breath to help you focus on less responsive areas of your body. To breathe in concert with the movements, pick a hand or foot with which to coordinate your breath. As that hand or foot moves up, you inhale. As it moves down, you exhale.

Try not to hold your breath at any time; let it smoothly shift from inhale to exhale and vice versa. For example, as your hand smoothly turns over near the front of your shoulder, let your breath smoothly and steadily move from inhale to exhale. As your hand circles from the outside of your foot to the inside, let your breath change smoothly from exhale to inhale.

Choose to coordinate your breath with the part of your body that you'd like to awaken. For example, if your left leg or foot seems like the least responsive part of your body, then breathe in concert with the movement of your left foot. If it is your right shoulder, then breathe in concert with the movement of your right hand.

## Emphasize the Downward Movement

A slightly more advanced aspect of Chi Balancing is to try to balance the up and down flows of energy between your body and the earth. The best way to do this is to emphasize the downward action of your hands and heels. The way chi works in the body is that if you can cause energy to sink down your body into the earth, chi will naturally rise up again. (This does not necessarily work in reverse; an upward flow won't necessarily cause a downward flow to occur.)

So in the Chi Balancing exercise you should play with sinking energy out of whichever heel is dropping at any time. You can simultaneously also play with moving chi with your falling hand down the front of your torso and the outside of your leg into the earth.

It is best to master the downward flow before trying to work with the upward flow. Once you get those downward movements going, then you start to play as well with the hand and foot that are rising. Try to move in such a way that you feel your dropping hand and heel causing your other hand and heel to rise up your body.

# CHAPTER 19

# Heart Opening

The Heart Opening exercise transfers energy between the left and right sides of your upper body. As this occurs, chi moves across your heart and your middle tantien or chakra, the center of your consciousness. This movement helps to open your heart to vitality, peace, compassion and balance.

## OVERVIEW

The continuous side-to-side motion of the arms and shoulder blades, together with the turning of your head, gently energizes your chi. It simultaneously frees up chi blockages in the important acupuncture points and meridians that control the functions of the heart. This improves circulation and helps to heal the heart muscle and the pericardium, the fibrous membrane surrounding the heart, as well as attached portions of the main blood vessels.

The movement loosens the whole upper body and increases the flexibility of the shoulder blades. This improves blood flow to the area, which helps to reduce or eliminate neck and shoulder pain. Your arms and hands gain greater strength and mobility. Your head is able to turn more easily, which is particularly important for older people, especially when driving.

This exercise is taught in three steps. Devote the time that you have available in your Chi Rev Workout for this exercise to practicing Step 1 until you feel very comfortable with it. Then practice Step 2 until it feels natural and easy. Finally practice Step 3.

## STEP 1: FOOT, LEG AND TORSO MOVEMENT— THE "SLOSH"

The foot and leg movements of the Heart Opening exercise are essentially the same as the leg movements of the Chi Balancing exercise, with one important exception.

In the Chi Balancing exercise you shift your weight and move your knees to lift and lower your heels. Your primary emphasis is moving your heels up and down and your knees forward and back.

In the Heart Opening exercise you move your legs and shift your weight in the same movement pattern. Here your primary emphasis is on the feeling of shifting your weight from side to side *(Figure 1)*.

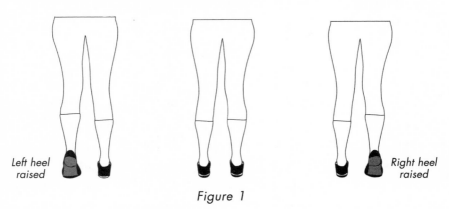

Left heel raised

Right heel raised

*Figure 1*

1. Begin to practice the leg and foot movements that you learned in the Chi Balancing exercise. Find a comfortable, slow rhythm and practice until your legs are warmed up and your movement begins to feel smooth, liquid and effortless.

2. Now focus on feeling your side-to-side weight shifts. Try to maintain your hips at the same height and feel them—and your torso and shoulders on top of them—move very stably in each direction.

For this exercise, it helps to think of your body as being composed of mostly water. In fact water comprises about sixty percent of your total body weight. Water is in your blood, your cells, your joints and even your bones.

When you move side to side try to feel as if all the water inside you—or the blood if you prefer—is washing back and forth from one side to the other. Let your legs, hips, torso, shoulders and head remain very stable as you move while allowing the water/blood inside you to "slosh" from side to side. The action is similar to when you hold a glass and move it gently from side to side; the glass itself moves as one piece while the water "sloshes" from side to side inside the glass.

3. Play with this leg and hip movement until you find a very comfortable, slow and steady rhythm. You should feel a gentle and relaxing transfer of blood, other fluids and chi from one side of your body to the other through your hips, belly, heart and even your brain.

## STEP 2. ADD ARM MOVEMENTS TO FURTHER AWAKEN AND OPEN YOUR HEART

The arm and hand motions of the Heart Opening exercise are relatively simple.

When moving your hands along your body or arms, try to keep your hands and fingers 6–8 inches away from your skin at all times.

**Beginning position:** *The standing posture you learned in the Chi Scanning exercise—face forward, feet flat on the floor, parallel to each other, approximately shoulder's width apart, with your weight distributed evenly on both feet.*

1. Slowly lift your arms and with your hands trace the energy pathways that are located along the outsides of your legs from your foot to your knee to your hip *(Figure 2A)*. Imagine you are pulling energy up the outsides of your legs.

2. Continue to raise your arms and trace your hands up the sides of your torso to your armpits and then to the front of your shoulders *(Figure 2B)*. Your desired motion is similar to what you would do if you were tickling yourself up along the sides of your ribs.

3. Extend your arms out to the sides of your body and trace with your fingertips along the insides of your upper arms, elbows, forearms and wrists *(Figure 2C)*. Use each hand to trace out along its own arm. As you move your arms out to the sides, progressively curve your wrists and fingers to keep your fingers pointing at the insides of your arms. Imagine you are pulling energy out along your arms to your hands.

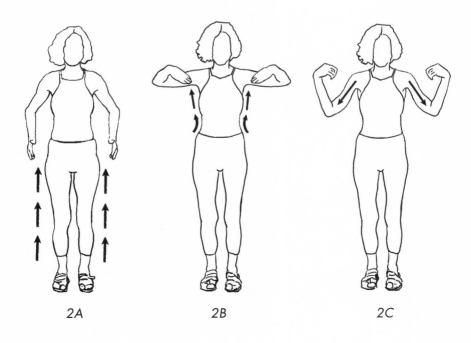

2A                              2B                              2C

**4.** When you've extended your arms and curled your fingers as far as is comfortable for you, then touch the tip of each thumb to the fingertips of each hand and turn your fingers so that they point downward *(Figure 2D)*. Each of your hands now has formed what we call a "beak hand" with all four fingertips lightly touching the tip of your thumb. If forming a beak hand is a strain for you with either hand, then only bring your fingertips as close to the tip of your thumb as is comfortable.

**5.** Open your hands and push your palms outward away from your sides, fingers pointing upward *(Figure 2E)*. Your arms are at the height of your shoulders or heart and your elbows are halfway bent and pointing downwards. If this position is in any way uncomfortable for you, then lower your arms slightly, bend your elbows a little more and move your arms forward and down until you are comfortable.

You are now ready to begin coordinating the hands and feet on both sides.

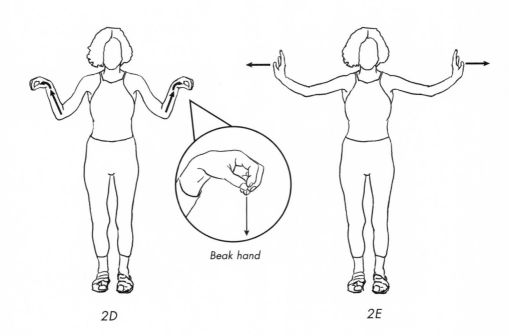

*Beak hand*

2D                                                                          2E

**6.** Move to one side *(Figure 3)*. Smoothly shift all your weight to one leg and lift your other heel.

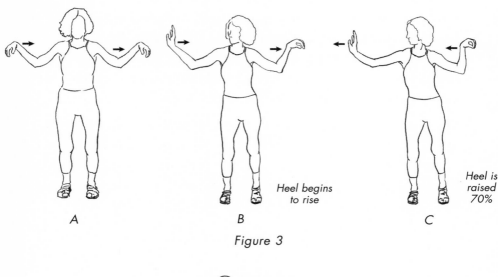

A                    B                    C

Heel begins
to rise

Heel is
raised
70%

*Figure 3*

## OVERVIEW

While you shift weight, your beak hand will be pulling in energy and the palm hand will be pushing it out. As this happens, energy will pass through the heart as a wave.

When you shift weight, the next movements should happen in a continuous flow.

Form a beak hand with the same hand that is on the side of your unweighted foot.

- ○ Bend that wrist as far as is comfortable.
- ○ Bend that elbow as far as is comfortable.
- ○ Slightly close your armpit, and if it is comfortable for you, slide your shoulder blade a little toward your spine.

Slightly extend the arm with the palm facing out.

- ○ Gently turn your head to look in the direction that you are moving, staying within your seventy percent range of motion.

- ○ If it is comfortable for you, slide your shoulder blade, on the side where your palm extends out, a little away from your spine and slightly open your armpit.
- ○ Unbend that elbow until it is extended two-thirds as far as your maximum range of motion.
- ○ Extend your wrist two-thirds as far as you can.
- ○ Open your palm as far as you can comfortably and let your fingers point upward, without straightening them fully.

Imagine you are steadily pushing energy out of your palm sideways for a couple of seconds.

Ideally, you will finish your weight shift (slosh) at the same time that you finish opening your palm. One arm is partially extended; the other is bent and has a beak hand. Your head and eyes are looking at the hand with the palm facing out.

## About the Shoulder Blades

Ideally, the shoulder blades will eventually move your arms in this exercise *(Figure 4)*.

The shoulder blade, on the side of the arm that is extending outward with your palm, moves away from the spine while the shoulder

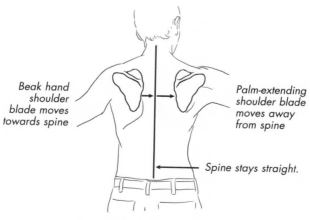

Beak hand shoulder blade moves towards spine

Palm-extending shoulder blade moves away from spine

Spine stays straight.

*Shoulder Blades as You Move Right*
*Figure 4*

blade connected to the retracting arm with the beak hand moves toward the spine. At first the shoulder blades will feel "locked up," but will gradually loosen if you practice in a very relaxed manner.

**7.** Move to the other side *(Figure 5)*. Repeat Instruction 6 as you shift and move toward the other side. Try to feel as if you generate the movement of your whole body from your leg.

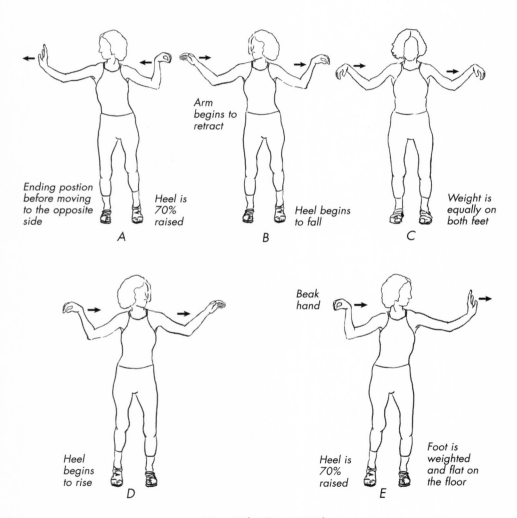

Arm begins to retract

Ending postion before moving to the opposite side

Heel is 70% raised

Heel begins to fall

Weight is equally on both feet

A                     B                     C

Heel begins to rise

Beak hand

Heel is 70% raised

Foot is weighted and flat on the floor

D                            E

*Move to the Opposite Side*

*Figure 5*

Try to keep your movements relaxed. Only lift your arms as high as is comfortable. Your shoulders should not rise or tighten.

**8.** Repeat moving from side to side and let your upper body relax and open. As you go back and forth from one side to the other, try to generate the movement of your whole body, including your arms, from your leg. Let your arms relax and move very fluidly. If you feel tension building anywhere in your body—especially your neck or shoulders—then slow down a bit, and extend and/or retract the appropriate arm a little less to help let go of your tension.

The goal of this exercise is to allow your upper body, especially your shoulders and neck and ultimately your heart, to relax and open. So don't worry about what you look like or how far you can stretch or reach. Only be concerned with how you feel.

Can you find a relaxed, liquid quality of movement where everything from your hips to your neck feels as if it lets go and flows in waves from side to side? Can you find a way of sloshing side to side that makes your whole upper body feel more alive and full of chi?

When you first begin practicing this step, it is a good idea to move your hands, arms, shoulders and neck in the sequential fashion described in Instruction 6. Once you have a good feel for how to move each part of your upper body in sequence, then your goal becomes moving all those parts simultaneously. When you have developed some skill practicing this way, you will feel that every part of your body is moving fluidly and continuously.

## STEP 3: COORDINATE BREATHING WITH THE MOVEMENTS

Now breathe in unison with the movements, using the principles of breathing that you learned in the Longevity Breathing exercise. As you move in one direction, inhale for eighty percent of your arm movements. Exhale during the last twenty percent of the movement, with the final extension of your palm and retraction of your beak hand.

Try to let the sloshing of your legs and hips from side to side power the movement of your whole body, including your arms and your breath. Play with how you do this movement with the goal of allowing your whole upper body to relax, release and open to the movement of chi back and forth across your body. With practice and over time, your heart can gradually open to greater vitality, and in turn, peace, compassion and balance.

## HOW THIS EXERCISE CAN HELP YOU AT WORK

If you're in front of your computer, or working at your desk, you can do this Heart Opening exercise sitting in your chair. While practicing:

- ○ Maintain the same body alignments that you had in the Chi Scanning exercise (except that your weight will shift and your head will move).
- ○ Let the heel of each foot go up and down as you move from side to side.
- ○ Move your hips from side to side to get the "sloshing" action, just as you would do if you were practicing the movement standing up.
- ○ When you are moving your head from side to side, try to look out into the distance. Gazing through a window is best.

If you do Heart Opening for about a minute or so every hour or half hour, it can help you:

- ○ Prevent stress from accumulating.
- ○ Improve your concentration and productivity.
- ○ Mitigate carpal tunnel syndrome and repetitive strain injuries.
- ○ Alleviate eyestrain.

The Chi Balancing exercise can also be done sitting to bring you some of these benefits. Working at a computer tends to induce shallow breathing. Longevity Breathing and Chi Scanning can counteract this, and are also very useful for reducing stress.

When you feel stress beginning to accumulate in the mid-morning or afternoon, if you can get up and take a break to do the whole Chi Rev Workout, it could make your workday much more relaxed and productive.

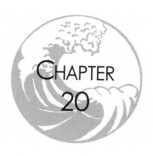

CHAPTER
20

# Freeing Trapped Chi

One benefit of all chi gung practices is to develop positive habits that become reflexive in all situations, including emergencies. The Freeing Trapped Chi exercise teaches you to instantaneously release the chi of your whole body into the ground. Doing so leads to:

○ Rapid discharge of stagnant or stuck, dead energy in your body.
○ Complete and immediate relaxation of your entire body.
○ A sense of becoming extremely grounded and stable.
○ A sense of your body and emotions becoming more balanced.

This move is extremely beneficial in many common disturbing situations—a traumatic emotional situation, such as an argument with someone at home or at work, an experience of fear or a sudden death in the family. When you have emotional trauma your internal dialogue speeds up as chi gets progressively more stuck in the head. You relive many of the memories associated with the trauma, remember every word spoken and repeat thoughts you might have used or wished you had said, over and over again. The solution lies in getting the chi out of your head and back into your body where it belongs. This is a specialty of the Freeing Trapped Chi exercise.

Likewise, this move is equally useful if your body goes into shock following an accident or a natural disaster, such as an earthquake or hurricane. During shock, the brain has more energy than it can handle and shuts down, causing hysteria or disorientation. In the West, a common method for bringing people out of hysteria is to slap them to bring them to their senses. However, this may cause a worsening of the problem because it can cause even more energy to get stuck in the head. Slapping someone can induce even more extreme paralysis.

In the chi practices of the East, the common method for bringing people out of hysteria is to lift the person and bring them down hard on their heels, hit their heels or have them stomp their feet. Chi energy suddenly drops down the body and releases so the brain and natural bodily functions can return to normal. The Freeing Trapped Chi exercise does the same.

## OVERVIEW

This is a primary "let go" movement, something which many who live in industrial and technologically driven societies have a hard time doing. Your main goal while doing the movement is to coordinate the dropping of your heels and a downward flick of your fingers, so that your energy lets go and drops in a sudden, but relaxed, manner into the ground. This may seem counterintuitive at first. With time, practice and the more relaxed you become, the more power, spring and speed you will gain in your release.

As your energy moves downward, stagnant energy is powerfully released from your kidneys, boosting your immune system and in turn allowing chi to rise upward from the earth and become balanced throughout your body.

This exercise is taught in three steps. Devote the time that you have available in your Chi Rev Workout for this exercise to practicing Step 1 until you feel very comfortable with it. Then practice Step 2, until it feels natural and easy. Finally, practice Step 3.

## Step 1:  Release Chi with Your Feet and Legs

**Beginning position:** *The standing posture you learned in the Chi Scanning exercise—face forward, feet flat on the floor, parallel to each other, approximately shoulder's width apart, with your weight distributed evenly on both feet.*

**1.** Very slowly rock forward onto the balls of your feet, lift your heels off the floor and press the balls of your feet strongly into the ground. Putting physical pressure on the ball of the foot causes energy to rise in the body. Do not raise your heels beyond seventy percent of your range of motion *(Figure 1)*. If you feel your foot vibrate or your foot or ankle tighten up, then you have gone too far. Lift your heels in as relaxed a fashion as possible.

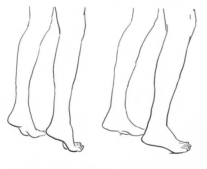

*70% of your range of motion for raising your heels might be somewhere between the two positions in this diagram*

*You might rise to 50% or even less, depending on personal circumstances*

*Freeing Trapped Chi Exercise: Heels Rise*
*Figure 1*

**2.** Suddenly drop your heels. The sudden pressure of the drop through your heels will cause energy from your entire body and legs to move downward and exit your feet. It is the suddenness and speed of the drop, not the power of your stomp, that maximizes the clearing of stagnant energy from your legs.

When you drop, allow your body to find a position that is completely relaxed. You feel all your joints have an internal bounce. As best as you can, drop your heels in such a way as to avoid stiffening, locking or feeling energy getting stuck inside any of your joints. You should feel the shock wave—from your heels suddenly landing—go smoothly through your whole body. This gently shakes your system to dislodge stagnant energy from your belly and your middle and lower back (where your kidneys are located) through your waist, legs and feet into the ground.

Ideally, you will make no noise when you drop your heels, like a cat that makes no noise when it pounces.

**3.** Best surfaces to practice on are grass, dirt, carpet and wood. Concrete is not recommended.

**4.** If your body is weak, you are ill, or if you have a back, leg or other injury, avoid counterproductive and unnecessary shock or harm to yourself by initially lifting your heels less than an inch off the ground and then very gently dropping them. Try to practice on as soft a surface as possible.

Repeat these movements until you can do them while keeping your body relaxed and your legs springy.

## Step 2: Release Chi with Your Hands and Arms

In this exercise, your hands will trace what is called the great meridian, which is located just under your skin, a few inches or so below your belly button. Known in Chinese as the dai mai, the great meridian encircles the entire torso, front to back *(Figure 2)*.

Directly connected to the great meridian, but deep in the core of your torso at this height, is your lower tantien, the most important energetic center in your body with respect to your physical health. All the energy lines of your body pertaining to physical health and well-being connect here.

Also on the great meridian, located on your spine directly behind the lower tantien is another important energy point, called mingmen, the door of life.

Mingmen is called the door of life because it is directly associated with the kidneys, internal organs that are the source of the body's chi or life-force energy. The lower tantien and mingmen are connected by an energy channel inside your body. Think of the lower tantien as the center of a horizontal wheel and the great meridian as the outside of the wheel. The great meridian connects all the vertical acupuncture lines in the body and transfers energy among them.

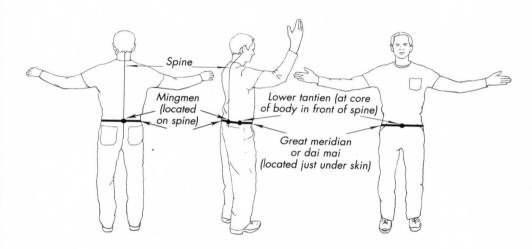

Lower Tantien, Mingmen and Great Meridian (Dai Mai)
Figure 2

**Beginning position:** *Stand with your feet shoulder's width apart and parallel, fingers pointing to the insides of your feet (Figure 3A).*

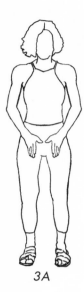

During the whole movement your palms will face your body. Your goal is to coordinate the sudden dropping of your heels with the flick of your hands and fingers.

1. Inhale and slowly and gradually raise your heels while your fingers simultaneously:

   a. Trace up the energy pathways of the inside of your legs to your thighs *(Figure 3B)* to the front of your hips and the front of your lower tantien *(Figure 3C)*.

   b. Trace the great meridian. Each of your palms circle back around the side of your waist as far toward your lower spine as you can maintain your comfort level *(Figures 3D, E & F)*. Ideally, your palms face mingmen on your spine, but your hands do not touch.

   c. Trace forward from mingmen along the great meridian to the lower tantien, gradually forming beak hands, as you did in the Chi Opening exercise. Finish forming them just as you reach the front of your torso and the lower tantien, at which your fingers should point *(Figure 3G & H)*. At this point, your heels should be raised to their highest level.

3A

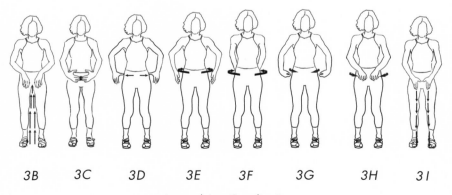

3B          3C          3D          3E          3F          3G          3H          3I

*Leg and Arm Coordination*

**2.** Simultaneously, flick your fingers toward the ground, exhale all your breath and suddenly drop your heels *(Figure 3I)*. Imagine that you are releasing chi from your palms and your fingertips straight down into the ground. The dropping action naturally will direct energy down the outsides of your legs.

During the flick, your hands should be as soft, pliable and springy as possible. The release of stagnant energy comes from the speed, not the physical power of the release.

○ As you flick, generate the feeling of releasing and throwing away energy from your armpits as well as your hands. The energy movement originates in the armpits and finishes by being expressed out through the fingers.
○ Tensing your fingers or putting overt physical strength in the flick will diminish its benefits. Speed is important, not power.

Let your fingers point toward the insides of your feet. You are now ready to bring energy back up again *(Figure 3J)*.

Repeat Instructions 1 and 2 in a continuous loop.

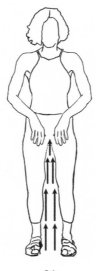

*3J*

## Step 3: Release Chi with Your Legs, Arms and Breath

1. Inhale slowly and steadily while you raise your hands and trace your palms up your inner leg to the front of your body at the height of your great meridian.

2. Exhale as you circle your hands along the great meridian around to your lower back.

3. Inhale as your hands return along the great meridian to the lower tantien.

4. Rapidly exhale in unison with the flick and the dropping of your heels in a very relaxed manner. The speed and relaxation of your exhale are the key here, not power.

### Important Points to Remember

The Freeing Trapped Chi exercise is about letting go. When you practice, recall an image of a kitten pouncing, flicking its paw or breathing. It remains completely relaxed and soft, seemingly without tension.

The exercise's primary purpose is to release stagnant energy. Since tension locks such energy into your system:

- Try to rise on the balls of your feet in such a way that you do not stiffen your feet, hips, legs or ankles.
- Remember that steady pressure on the balls of your feet causes chi to rise up your body while pressure on your heels causes chi to drop.
- To stay balanced, if you need to, rather than gradually lifting your heals, slowly move your weight from your heels to the balls of your feet. As you move your arms and only just before the flick, actually raise your heels off the ground.
- Try not to hold your breath, even for a microsecond.
- Just let go when you drop your heels, flick and suddenly exhale; don't push.

The Freeing Trapped Chi exercise is an interesting challenge in many ways. Initially, the difficulty lies in coordinating your arms, legs and breath. Later you focus on how well you can just release, and relax and soften your arms and hands when you flick and drop. This is not easy and most of us develop this skill only very gradually.

One key is to feel as if the rise of your heels and hands occurs very slowly and lightly and is powered by a sense that your body just fills up with energy. Maybe the image of a balloon filling up with helium is helpful.

Another key is that when you drop, you instantaneously release all your energy through your arms and legs and out with your breath—as if you were a balloon that has just been popped.

Remember, the more you release, the more you will relax; and the more you relax, the more you will release.

## Learning to Feel Chi Is a Gradual Process

Don't worry if you can't feel your chi at first. Some people might take months or even years to develop a strong sense of their own chi. The Chi Rev Workout will get your chi moving even if you aren't aware of it. The ability to feel may come and go in a peek-a-boo, now you see it, now you don't manner. You may start to feel a sense of pressure, buzzing or electricity in your hands as you do the movements. Over time as you continue to practice, your awareness of chi will become more comprehensive and precise.

CHAPTER
21

# Nothing Left to Do But to Do It

There is an old Taoist saying, "The teacher leads you to the gate, but only you, by your own effort, can pass through." Whether you have tried some of the elements of the Chi Rev Workout or you are taking a class in any kind of chi practice, at the most basic level, you need to start somewhere. Then it becomes a relatively small daily effort to set a time and adopt a regular rhythm in your life that includes your practice.

Chi practices are as important and essential to us as sleep, food and water. One of the hardest lessons in life is to learn how to nourish ourselves. Perhaps this book has helped you understand the importance of cultivating your chi. While many of us take time to nurture others with positive energy or caretaking, we often neglect our inner worlds. We disregard the connection—within us and all around us—that keeps us balanced and alive. We lose the ability to feel our chi. The Chi Revolution is asking you to step through the gate.

## SUSTAINABLE PRACTICE

Where do you start? You start with what you can do right now, right this minute. You will only have success with what you can stand to do, what you grow to love—exercises you can actually do, not what you *should* do. Taking one small step toward yourself right now will encourage you to take others. It will give you a foundation upon which to build. You will find it becomes increasingly easier to move from the basics you can do right now to the more advanced practices available to you.

Right now, take three breaths and use them as a measure of how you breathe. Or take three breaths and allow the breath to help you consciously relax. Slowly, you could build up to the four minutes of breathing suggested in the Chi Rev Workout. Maybe you could try the Chi Balancing exercise for five to ten repetitions. It takes under a minute and gets your breathing practice in as well. There is nothing like killing two birds with one stone.

If you start with one minute here, two minutes there, five minutes there, the effect on your nerves and chi is cumulative. You do not have to start by doing everything all at once and, in fact, it is not recommended. Your practice outlook should be a positive one, and doing too much too soon is a sure-fire strategy for failure. Your practice has to be sustainable. The point is, start somewhere right now. Something is better than nothing. Even if you are only doing a few minutes here and there each day, you are supporting your choice to nourish yourself and your chi.

## CLASSES

The easiest way to establish a chi practice is in a class setting with an instructor who can teach you the movements and the principles behind them. Instructors can also give you caveats to avoid injury. Most importantly, classes help establish a rhythm of learning and practice. When we were children, we had classes in ballet, soccer, creative writing, painting, sewing, swimming, chess or football. Classes were usually held at the same time and days of the week, and we were conditioned to learn and practice at these times. We did not have to think much about the commitment because we just showed up at the set time without all the intellectual nonsense about when, why or how. The same will hold true for you now. Lessons are not only about developing a skill set; they are also about social interaction and coming together with others who share our interests and support each other. When a group does chi practices together, the collective energy is raised and will help to lift you and carry you along with it.

If classes don't work for you, use training guides such as books, DVDs and CDs. I have spent a great deal of my time in the last few years producing materials that will help you learn from the comfort of your living room because experience has taught me that establishing a practice rhythm is so important. If you choose to learn on your own, be sure to designate a time and place just as you would for a class.

## SET YOURSELF UP FOR SUCCESS BY NOT LEAVING PRACTICING TO CHANCE

If you think a skill is worth having, the fact is that, with practice, all you can do is get better. Even though you might be capable of learning basic movements from a retreat, weekend workshop or video, it takes time for the movements to work deeply in your body, emotions and mind. If you practice, you will feel how the exercises begin to change you on both gross and subtle levels.

As with any skill you develop, you first have to be willing to apply the beginner's mentality—repetition, getting feedback from those who already have the ability, building on easy successes and advancing only when you have the basics down pat. Nobody starts out being great, or even competent, in a day. When John Lennon started composing songs, he knew he had a passion and some talent. He put in the time and practice to develop his talent into the great songwriter he became. The same is true for internal chi exercises. Nobody starts by doing them perfectly. The experts will tell you that perfection is unreachable, a trait that is only reserved for gods.

I once asked my greatest teacher Liu Hung Chieh, "Have you ever done tai chi perfectly?" He said that one day after decades of practicing he thought he had. But then, he said, it was several weeks later when he suddenly realized he had done tai chi even better than the time before. Who knows how many times this happened.

Only a fool says, "Well, I have to eat three healthy meals a day and if I don't, I'm not going to eat at all." If you want to live in the real world with that attitude, get ready to starve. The perfectionist's outlook for the vast majority is a failure's strategy. Maybe if you are very wealthy you can take three hours a day to eat extremely well; however, most of us have to make compromises from time to time because it is the best we can do. Enough is enough. The same principle applies to establishing a time to practice. For many, there will be no perfect situation, no perfect time to start nor a perfect place or circumstance.

The good news is that chi exercises can be done virtually anywhere, anytime—standing, sitting or even lying down. By harnessing the power of your chi, you take back control of your health and manage your stress so you are vital and energized for your life. Establishing a regular rhythm of practice is a big step. It will be worth it to you when you can look back and see how far you have come. Without your health you cannot take pleasure in anything.

## CARVING OUT PRACTICE TIME

Whether you take a class or decide to learn chi practices from a DVD or a book, you need to carve out some time in your daily schedule that makes sense to you. If you are a disciplined person, this will be relatively easy for you, provided you place some value on it. If not, setting a regular practice time, even for three to five minutes a couple of times each day, will make a tremendous difference for your long-term progress. Maybe take a few deep breaths when you become aware of negative self-talk, for example. In only a few minutes you will enable your nervous system to slow down, relax and allow your chi to flow uninhibited. Practicing regularly will benefit you more than not doing any chi practice during the week and trying to make up for it on the weekend. A little consistency is better than overdoing it every once in awhile. Observe the seventy percent rule. Not overdoing your practice makes it easier to stick to it without trying to talk yourself out of it.

The best time to practice is sometime, rather than never. Maybe you find it easiest to practice in the morning when you first wake up; maybe you find it easier just after the kids go to bed. By starting with only that small regular rhythm, just those few minutes, you will most likely, and virtually effortlessly, start extending your practice a few minutes here and there. As you reinforce positive rhythms, they will physically solidify in the brain, recondition the body and powerfully strengthen and cultivate your chi.

## FIFTEEN MINUTES TO FREEDOM

Once you establish a regular rhythm of practice, you will want to slowly and easily extend it to fifteen to twenty minutes of continuous practice to achieve basic health and relaxation benefits. From a purely physical point of view, it takes the body about that many minutes for the chi to really get going and for the blood to fully engorge the blood vessels enough to make a significant difference. It is the same for any cardiovascular exercise.

Don't practice for a long time two hours before you plan to go to sleep. Chi exercises can wake you up more than any caffeine. The exceptions are TAO yoga or Chi Scanning, which help calm you down and bring you to a still point.

## ESTABLISHING POSITIVE INNER RHYTHMS

Before any new practice can take hold inside you, a rhythm must be established in your body and central nervous system. Most people have deeply established rhythms: when they get up, eat, go to work, exercise. Integrating novel aspects into your rhythms is often difficult because the neural pathways and the corresponding highly reinforced, conditioned responses in the body require reprogramming. Your brain and body will need time to make the new physical connections. Each time you practice, however, you are strengthening these pathways so that you no longer have to think about what to do—you just do it.

Rhythms are established by repeatedly activating neural pathways in the brain, whether positive or negative. Chemical reactions in the brain, or neurotransmitters, reinforce positive or negative rhythms. In many people, habits of self-neglect and negative patterns accumulate over long periods. One of those patterns is deep resistance to change. Many people find it difficult to reestablish healthier flows, particularly with regard to diet or exercise. A common excuse is "I don't have time." What that usually indicates is the old conditioning of the brain taking over to suppress the need to evolve and change.

Whether you are learning in a class or on your own, it takes anywhere from three weeks to a month for your body to accustom itself to new practices and to have them take hold at the cellular level. Then, chi practices become as natural and important as eating or brushing your teeth. In other words, a positive feedback loop is created, kicking in to help you maintain them when you meet internal or external resistance.

## THE BEST CHI PRACTICE

Many of my students ask me, "Is there a best chi practice?" To some extent, the answer depends on your own personal preferences. That said, if there were only one thing I could do to help you, I would teach you to breathe properly. No matter what you do, breathing continuously and smoothly is paramount.

One of the great benefits of chi practices is that there is enough variety for you to find a practice that works for you. There are hundreds of chi gung movements, five major tai chi styles, three internal martial arts, TAO yoga, partner exercises, sitting and standing practices—whatever your personal preference, you can find a method that suits you. They all effectively and systematically improve health, relax the body to mitigate stress and strengthen your chi.

## CHI PRACTICES ARE LIFE TOOLS

Chi has the power to grow and strengthen inside you exponentially. After a certain amount of practice, which differs for everyone, the effects take hold and begin growing ever more quickly inside you. A small snowball grows into a large one as it rolls downhill, gathering momentum, size and strength. Likewise, investing $1,000 earns a little interest at first, but after some years the interest and principle compounds and becomes $10,000.

Although chi practices are great for cultivating health and well-being, they can also be used when you have to deal with difficult situations. Maybe you know you're going to face a tense situation at work or at home. Maybe the traffic is a nightmare, day after day. Maybe you're sitting at your computer and you feel the strain building up in your hands and arms. When the internal chatter starts running in circles, havoc soon follows in your head, stomach and shoulder muscles. This is the moment to start taking conscious breaths and focusing on relaxing and letting go. Release any blockages before they have time to bind inside you and create more trouble. Get up and do whatever chi movement exercise you know to get the chi flowing again.

# The Magic of Chi

The power of chi is deeply transformative. Nourishing your chi will make you healthier and more relaxed for the rest of your life, well into old age. Chi work clears the physical blockages and negative emotions and thoughts, bringing back the joy and spontaneity you had as a child. More advanced chi practices will help you connect strongly to yourself and will allow genuine love and compassion for yourself and others to flow naturally. As you open up to your human potential, the deep positive rhythms of the universe will come to your aid.

Chi practices can inspire you for the rest of your life. One of the most magical qualities I have found is that they continue to interest, engage and teach me new lessons, even after four decades of daily practice. They can do the same for you. If you could choose to have more external or inner wealth, consider that an inner exploration to harness the chi flowing inside and through you is a true path to inner peace and happiness. It is something that no external object could ever offer for more than a few fleeting moments.

The Chi Revolution is about an awakening, from deep within, starting with you. Will *you* go through the gate?

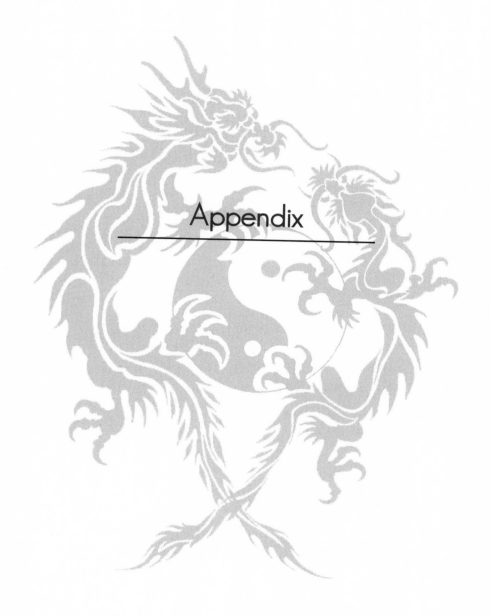

# Appendix

# Taoism: A Living Tradition

M any traditions based on ancient philosophies and religions have vibrantly continued into modern times. Since they manifest in our lives today they are commonly referred to as living traditions. These include Christianity, Islam, Judaism, Buddhism, Vedanta and Taoism. The latter three actively practice physical exercises and energy work.

Taoism is the least known of the living traditions. Although its main literary works—the *I Ching,* the writings of Chuang Tse and the *Tao Te Ching* by Lao Tse—are well known and available in many translations, the practical methods and techniques of implementing Taoist philosophy in daily life are little documented in the West.

One branch of living Taoist philosophy is about developing and using one's personal chi or life-force energy to strengthen, heal and benefit oneself and others. This branch encompasses two broad traditions: water and fire. The Water method, passed down by Lao Tse over 2,500 years ago, emphasizes effort without force, relaxation and letting go, as the flow of water slowly erodes rock. The Fire method, developed 1,500 years later, emphasizes force, pushing forward and breaking through barriers.

The Taoist lineages that Bruce Frantzis holds are in the Water tradition, which has received little exposure in the West. Part of his lineage empowers and directs him to bring practices based on that tradition to Westerners. He learned the Chinese language and became immersed in the traditions of China during more than a decade of training there.

What is known from the *Tao Te Ching, I Ching* and other Taoist texts is almost entirely literary. While Frantzis learned with his main teacher, Grandmaster Liu Hung Chieh, texts were presented as: "This is what they say; this is what they mean; this is how to do them." Frantzis offers an unprecedented bridge to this pragmatic approach to spirituality as we are not aware of any other English or European language source for which this style of teaching exists. It means that spirituality is not just an aspiration for which people strive in the dark, "in a mirror, darkly," to quote St. Paul, but it becomes a genuine, accomplishable reality.

# The Frantzis
# Energy Arts® System

D rawing on sixteen years of training in Asia, Bruce Frantzis has developed a practical, comprehensive system of programs that can enable people of all ages and fitness levels to increase their core energy and attain vibrant health.

## Opening the Energy Gates of Your Body™ Chi Gung

This program introduces 3,000-year-old chi gung techniques that are fundamental to advancing any energy arts practice. Core exercises teach you the basic body alignments and methods for increasing your internal awareness of chi in your body and for dissolving blocked chi.

## Marriage of Heaven and Earth™ Chi Gung

This chi gung incorporates techniques widely used in China to help heal back, neck, spine and joint problems. It is especially effective for helping to mitigate injuries related to repetitive stress and carpal tunnel problems. This program teaches some important nei gung components, including openings and closings (pulsing), more complex breathing techniques and how to conciously move chi through the acupuncture meridians.

## Bend the Bow™ Spinal Chi Gung

Bend the Bow continues the work of strengthening and regenerating spine that is learned in the Marriage of Heaven and Earth chi gung. This program incorporates nei gung components for awakening and controlling the energies of the spine.

## Spiraling Energy Body™ Chi Gung

This advanced program teaches you to dramatically raise your energy level and master how energy moves in circles and spirals throughout your body. It incorporates nei gung components for directing the upward flow of energy; projecting chi along the body's spiraling pathways; delivering or projecting energy at will to or from any part of the body; and activating the body's left, right and central channels and the microcosmic orbit.

## Gods Playing in the Clouds™ Chi Gung

Gods Playing in the Clouds incorporates some of the oldest and most powerful Taoist rejuvenation techniques. This program amplifies all the physical, breathing and energetic components learned in earlier chi gung programs and completes the process of integrating all the components of nei gung. It is also the final stage of learning to strengthen and balance the energies of your three tantiens, central energy channel and spine. Gods Playing in the Clouds chi gung serves as a spiritual bridge to TAO meditation.

## Longevity Breathing® Program

Bruce Frantzis has developed this method to teach authentic Taoist breathing in six systematic stages—breathing from 1) the front of the belly; 2) the sides of the belly; 3) the lower back and kidneys; 4) the back of the lungs; 5) the top of the lungs; 6) the spine. Breathing with the whole body has been used for millennia to enhance the ability to dissolve and release energy blockages in the mind/body, enhancing well-being and spiritual awareness.

Incorporating these breathing techniques into any other Taoist energy practice will help bring out its full potential.

## Dragon and Tiger Medical Chi Gung

Ideal for beginners, Dragon and Tiger chi gung is one of the most direct and accessible low-impact chi gung healing methods originating from China. Frantzis learned this 1,500-year-old form of medical chi gung from a Chinese doctor. Dragon and Tiger activates the energy in your acupuncture meridians to help strengthen your immune system and make you healthier. The seven movements can be done by virtually anyone, whatever their state of health or fitness level.

## TAO Yoga

TAO yoga is ancient China's soft, yet powerful alternative to what is popularly known today as Hatha yoga. The primary emphasis in Frantzis' method of teaching TAO yoga is to stimulate the flow of chi and free up any blocked energy. Combining gentle postures and Longevity Breathing techniques systematically opens the body's energy channels thereby activating and stimulating chi flow. Postures are held from two to five minutes and require virtually no muscular effort, so they enable you to easily focus on what is internal so you can feel where the chi is blocked and gently free it up.

## TAO Meditation

Frantzis is a lineage holder in the gentle Water method of Taoist meditation passed down from the teachings of Lao Tse, one of China's most revered ancient sages, over 2,500 years ago. The art and power of Taoist meditation is not well known to Westerners and is often confused with Buddhist meditation. Bruce calls the technique he has developed TAO meditation. In the Taoist tradition, the road to spirituality involves more than obtaining health, calmness and a stable, peaceful mind. It includes using chi to help you release anxieties, expectations, mental churnings, conditionings and negative emotions—referred to as blockages—that prevent you from feeling truly alive and joyful. The first goal is to address spiritual responsibility for yourself, helping you become a relaxed, spontaneous, fully mature and open human being. A second goal is awakening the great human potential inside you, fostering compassion and balance. The third is reaching inner stillness—a place deep inside you that is absolutely permanent and stable.

## Tai Chi and Ba Gua as Health Arts

Tai chi and ba gua practiced as health arts intensify the benefits of the core chi gung practices.

## Internal Martial Arts

Rather  than using muscular tension or anger for power, the internal martial arts teach you to use relaxation, chi and stillness of mind to accomplish the pragmatic goal of winning in a violent confrontation.

### Tai Chi Chuan

Tai chi is a potent martial art. Frantzis trained extensively in the traditional Wu, Yang and Chen styles of tai chi chuan, including short and long forms, push hands, self-defense techniques and such traditional weapons as sticks and swords.

### Ba Gua Chang

Ba gua (also transliterated as *pa kua*) was designed to fight up to eight opponents at once. Virtually no other martial art system or style, internal or external, has combined and seamlessly integrated into one package the whole pantheon of martial arts fighting techniques as effectively as ba gua. Ba gua is first and foremost an art of internal energy movement that embodies the eight primal energies encompassed by the eight trigrams of the *I Ching*. The basic internal power training consists of learning eight palm changes and combining them with walking, spiraling and twisting arm movements as well as constant changes of direction.

## Hsing-I Chuan

Hsing-i (also transliterated as *xing yi*) emphasizes all aspects of the mind to create its forms and fighting movements. It is an equally potent healing practice because it makes people healthy and then very strong. Its five basic movements are related to the five primal elements or phases of energy—metal, water, wood, fire and earth—upon which Chinese medicine is based and from which all manifested phenomena are created. Hsing-i training is based on a linear, militaristic approach: marching in straight lines, with a powerful emphasis at the end of every technique on mentally or physically taking an enemy down.

# The Living Taoism Collection

## Books

As a longtime practitioner of Taoist energy arts, Bruce Frantzis teaches and writes books with deep gratitude to his main teacher, the late Taoist Lineage Master Liu Hung Chieh of Beijing, who so generously shared his knowledge of the TAO.

Other books in the Living Taoism™ collection include *Opening the Energy Gates of Your Body: Chi Gung for Lifelong Health; Tai Chi: Health for Life; The Power of Martial Arts and Chi: Combat and Energy Secrets of Ba Gua, Tai Chi and Hsing-I;* and two volumes on the Water method of TAO meditation, *Relaxing Into Your Being* and *The Great Stillness*.

The newest addition to the collection is *Dragon and Tiger Medical Chi Gung Instruction Manual* from which much of the Chi Rev Workout presented in this book was derived. The manual provides detailed instructions to practice each of the seven movements of Dragon and Tiger and is only available through EnergyArts.com.

# CDs and DVDs

Subjects range from a general introduction to Taoist practices to specific topics such as Opening the Energy Gates chi gung, tai chi self-defense techniques and Longevity Breathing®.

Featured is Frantzis' complete meditation course, *The TAO of Letting Go,* a six-CD set. For the first time in the West, he shares the Inner Dissolving method of TAO meditation. This special recording introduces you to how powerfully meditation can help you let go of tension, fear, anger and pain. Frantzis guides you through turning inwards to awaken the great human potential inside yourself and move closer to feeling alive and joyful.

Frantzis' recently released *Ancient Songs of the TAO* is a collection of never-before-recorded chants in ancient Chinese as a three-CD set. These Taoist liturgies are used to balance and transform the energetic frequencies within a human being.

## Training Opportunities

Bruce Frantzis is the founder of Energy Arts, Inc., based in Marin County, California. Energy Arts offers instructor certification programs, retreats and corporate and public workshops and lectures in North America and Europe. Bruce bridges the gap between Chinese culture and the West. He has taught Living Taoism to over 15,000 Westerners and certified over 300 instructors worldwide. Visit EnergyArts.com for details of events currently being offered.

## Instructor Certification

Prior training in Frantzis Energy Arts programs is a requirement for most instructor courses. The certification process is rigorous to ensure that instructors teach the authentic traditions inherent in these arts.

# Train with a Frantzis Energy Arts Certified Instructor

The Energy Arts Web site, EnergyArts.com, contains a directory of all the certified instructors worldwide. Since Frantzis no longer offers regular ongoing classes, he recommends locating an instructor in your area for regular training and for building on the teachings in his workshops and retreats.

## Contact Information

Energy Arts, Inc.
P.O. Box 99
Fairfax, CA 94978
415.454.5243

## We invite you to visit EnergyArts.com:

○ Sign up for our mailing list to receive notices from Bruce, including his newsletter, *ChiTalk*.
○ Receive the latest details on events and training materials.
○ Discover ways to join Bruce in addressing the health crisis.
○ See video clips of the chi gung and martial arts forms discussed in this book.
○ Find a certified instructor near you or learn how to become one.
○ Inquire about hosting a workshop or speaking engagement with Bruce.

# Bibliography

Chuang Tzu, *The Way of Chuang Tzu,* translated by Thomas Merton. Shambhala Publications, 2004.

Emoto, Masaru, *The Hidden Messages in Water.* Atria Books, a division of Simon & Schuster, Inc., 2005.

Fixx, Jim, *Complete Book of Running.* Random House, Inc., 1977.

*I Ching or Book of Changes:* The Richard Wilhelm Translation rendered into English by Cary F. Baynes. Bollingen Foundation, 1950.

Liao, Waysun, *T'ai Chi Classics.* Shambhala Publications, 2001.

Lao Tse (Lao Tzu), *The Tao Te Ching,* translated by Gia-Fu Feng and Jane English. Vintage, 2007.

Lipton, Bruce H., *The Biology of Belief: Unleashing the Power of Consciousness, Matter and Miracles.* Mountain of Love Productions and Elite Press, 2005.

McTaggart, Lynne, *The Intention Experiment: Using Your Thoughts to Change Your Life and the World.* Free Press, a division of Simon & Schuster, Inc., 2007.

McTaggart, Lynne, *The Field: The Quest for the Secret Force of the Universe.* Harper Paperbacks, an imprint of HarperCollins Publishers, 2003.

Zhuangzi (Chuang Tzu) *Zhuangzi: Basic Writings,* translated by Burton Watson. Columbia University Press, 2003.